I0223233

PLANT-BASED COOKBOOK

2022

DELICIOUS RECIPES FOR EATING WELL WITHOUT MEAT FOR BEGINNERS

PAUL VUOLO

Copyright 2022

All Rights Reserved

All rights reserved. No part of this book may be reproduced or copied in any form or by any means, electronic or mechanical, including photocopying, recording or by any information storage and retrieval system, without written permission from the publisher, except for the inclusion of brief quotations in a review.

Warning-Disclaimer

The aim of the information in this book is to be as accurate as possible. The author and publisher shall have neither liability or responsibility to anyone with respect to any loss or damage caused, or alleged to be caused, directly or indirectly by the information provided in this book.

Table of Contents

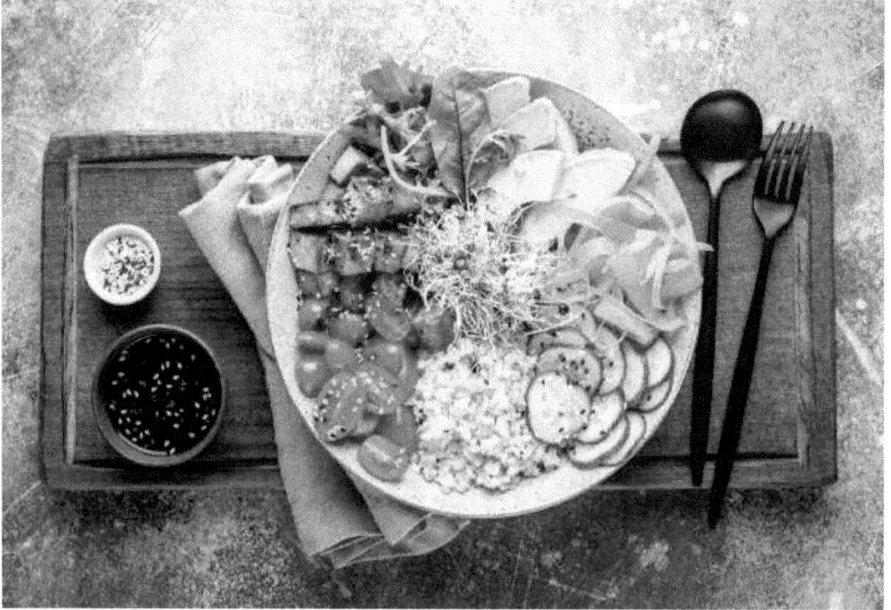

INTRODUCTION

It is only until recently that more and more people are starting to embrace the plant-based diet lifestyle. As to what exactly has drawn tens of millions of people into this lifestyle is debatable. However, there is growing evidence demonstrating that following a primarily plant-based diet lifestyle leads to better weight control and general health, free of many chronic diseases. What are the Health Benefits of a Plant-Based Diet? As it turns out, eating plant-based is one of the healthiest diets in the world. Healthy vegan diets include plenty of fresh products, whole grains, legumes, and healthy fats such as seeds and nuts. They are abundant with antioxidants, minerals, vitamins, and dietary fiber. Current scientific researches pointed out that higher consumption of plant-based foods is associated with a lower risk of mortality from conditions such as cardiovascular disease, type 2 diabetes, hypertension, and obesity. Vegan eating plans often rely heavily on healthy staples, avoiding animal products that are loaded with antibiotics, additives, and hormones. Plus, consuming a higher proportion of essential amino acids with animal protein can be damaging to human health. Since animal products contain much 8 more fat than plant-based foods, it's not a shocker that studies have shown that meat-eaters have nine times the obesity rate of vegans. This leads us to the next point, one of the greatest benefits of the vegan diet – weight loss. While many people choose to live a vegan life for ethical reasons, the diet itself can help you achieve your weight loss goals. If you're struggling to shift pounds, you may want to consider trying a plant-based diet. How exactly? As a vegan, you will reduce the number of high-calorie foods such as full-fat dairy products, fatty fish, pork and other cholesterol containing foods such as eggs. Try replacing such foods with high fiber and protein-rich alternatives that will keep you fuller longer. The key is focusing on nutrient-dense, clean and natural foods and avoid empty calories such as sugar, saturated fats, and highly processed foods. Here are a few tricks that help me maintain my weight on the vegan diet for years. I eat vegetables as a main course; I consume good fats in moderation – a good fat such as olive oil does not make you fat; I exercise regularly and cook at home. Enjoy!

Classic Barbecue Sauce

(Ready in about 5 minutes | Servings 20)

Per serving : Calories: 36; Fat: 0.3g; Carbs: 8.6g; Protein: 0.2g

Ingredients

1 cup brown sugar

1 cup ketchup

1/4 cup wine vinegar

1/3 cup water

1 tablespoon soy sauce

2 tablespoon mustard powder

1 teaspoon black pepper

2 teaspoons sea salt

Directions

Mix all the ingredients in your blender or food processor.

Blend until uniform and smooth.

Bon appétit!

Garden Herb Mustard

(Ready in about 35 minutes | Servings 10)

Per serving : Calories: 34; Fat: 1.6g; Carbs: 3.5g; Protein: 1.3g

Ingredients

1/2 cup mustard powder

5 tablespoons mustard seeds, ground

1/4 cup water

1/4 cup beer

2 tablespoons sherry vinegar

1 ½ teaspoons coarse sea salt

1 tablespoon agave syrup

1 tablespoon dried cilantro

1 tablespoon dried basil

Directions

Thoroughly combine the mustard powder, ground mustard seeds, water and beer in a mixing bowl; let it stand for about 30 minutes.

Add in the remaining ingredients and stir to combine well.

Let it sit at least 12 hours before serving. Bon appétit!

Classic Homemade Ketchup

(Ready in about 25 minutes | Servings 10)

Per serving : Calories: 24; Fat: 0g; Carbs: 5.5g; Protein: 0.5g

Ingredients

4 ounces canned tomato paste

2 tablespoons agave syrup

1/4 cup red wine vinegar

1/4 cup water

1/2 teaspoon kosher salt

1/4 teaspoon garlic powder

Directions

Preheat a saucepan over medium flame. Then, add all the ingredients to a saucepan and bring it to a boil.

Turn the heat to a simmer; let it simmer, stirring continuously, for about 20 minutes or until the sauce has thickened.

Store in a glass jar in your refrigerator. Bon appétit!

Cashew, Lime and Dill Sauce

(Ready in about 25 minutes | Servings 8)

Per serving : Calories: 24; Fat: 0g; Carbs: 5.5g; Protein: 0.5g

Ingredients

1 cup raw cashews

1/2 cup water

2 tablespoons dill

1 tablespoon lime juice

Sea salt and red pepper, to taste

Directions

Place all the ingredients in the bowl of your food processor or high-speed blender until smooth, uniform and creamy.

Season to taste and serve with crudités.

Ligurian Walnut Sauce

(Ready in about 30 minutes | Servings 4)

Per serving : Calories: 263; Fat: 24.1g; Carbs: 9g; Protein: 5.5g

Ingredients

1/2 cup almond milk

1 slice white bread, crusts removed

1 (about 50 halves) cup raw walnuts

1/2 teaspoon garlic powder

1 teaspoon onion powder

1 teaspoon smoked paprika

2 tablespoons olive oil

1 tablespoon basil, chopped

3 curry leaves

Sea salt and ground black pepper, to taste

Directions

Put the almond milk and bread in a bowl and let it soak well.

Transfer the soaked bread to the bowl of your food processor or high-speed blender; add in the remaining ingredients.

Process until smooth, uniform and creamy.

Serve with pasta or zucchini noodles. Bon appétit!

Chia, Maple and Dijon Sauce

(Ready in about 10 minutes | Servings 4)

Per serving : Calories: 126; Fat: 9g; Carbs: 8.3g; Protein: 1.5g

Ingredients

2 tablespoons chia seeds

5 tablespoons extra-virgin olive oil

1 ½ tablespoons maple syrup

2 teaspoons Dijon mustard

1 tablespoon red wine vinegar

Sea salt and ground black pepper, to taste

Directions

Put all the ingredients into a mixing bowl; whisk to combine and emulsify.

Let it sit for 15 minutes so the chia can expand. Bon appétit!

SOUPS & SALADS

Classic Lentil Soup with Swiss Chard

(Ready in about 25 minutes | Servings 5)

Per serving : Calories: 148; Fat: 7.2g; Carbs: 14.6g; Protein: 7.7g

Ingredients

2 tablespoons olive oil

1 white onion, chopped

1 teaspoon garlic, minced

2 large carrots, chopped

1 parsnip, chopped

2 stalks celery, chopped

2 bay leaves

1/2 teaspoon dried thyme

1/4 teaspoon ground cumin

5 cups roasted vegetable broth

1 ¼ cups brown lentils, soaked overnight and rinsed

2 cups Swiss chard, torn into pieces

Directions

In a heavy-bottomed pot, heat the olive oil over a moderate heat. Now, sauté the vegetables along with the spices for about 3 minutes until they are just tender.

Add in the vegetable broth and lentils, bringing it to a boil. Immediately turn the heat to a simmer and add in the bay leaves. Let it cook for about 15 minutes or until lentils are tender.

Add in the Swiss chard, cover and let it simmer for 5 minutes more or until the chard wilts.

Serve in individual bowls and enjoy!

Spicy Winter Farro Soup

(Ready in about 30 minutes | Servings 4)

Per serving : Calories: 298; Fat: 8.9g; Carbs: 44.6g; Protein: 11.7g

Ingredients

2 tablespoons olive oil

1 medium-sized leek, chopped

1 medium-sized turnip, sliced

2 Italian peppers, seeded and chopped

1 jalapeno pepper, minced

2 potatoes, peeled and diced

4 cups vegetable broth

1 cup farro, rinsed

1/2 teaspoon granulated garlic

1/2 teaspoon turmeric powder

1 bay laurel

2 cups spinach, turn into pieces

Directions

In a heavy-bottomed pot, heat the olive oil over a moderate heat. Now, sauté the leek, turnip, peppers and potatoes for about 5 minutes until they are crisp-tender.

Add in the vegetable broth, farro, granulated garlic, turmeric and bay laurel; bring it to a boil.

Immediately turn the heat to a simmer. Let it cook for about 25 minutes or until farro and potatoes have softened.

Add in the spinach and remove the pot from the heat; let the spinach sit in the residual heat until it wilts. Bon appétit!

Rainbow Chickpea Salad

(Ready in about 30 minutes | Servings 4)

Per serving : Calories: 378; Fat: 24g; Carbs: 34.2g; Protein: 10.1g

Ingredients

16 ounces canned chickpeas, drained

1 medium avocado, sliced

1 bell pepper, seeded and sliced

1 large tomato, sliced

2 cucumber, diced

1 red onion, sliced

1/2 teaspoon garlic, minced

1/4 cup fresh parsley, chopped

1/4 cup olive oil

2 tablespoons apple cider vinegar

1/2 lime, freshly squeezed

Sea salt and ground black pepper, to taste

Directions

Toss all the ingredients in a salad bowl.

Place the salad in your refrigerator for about 1 hour before serving.

Bon appétit!

Mediterranean-Style Lentil Salad

(Ready in about 20 minutes + chilling time | Servings 5)

Per serving : Calories: 348; Fat: 15g; Carbs: 41.6g; Protein: 15.8g

Ingredients

1 ½ cups red lentil, rinsed

1 teaspoon deli mustard

1/2 lemon, freshly squeezed

2 tablespoons tamari sauce

2 scallion stalks, chopped

1/4 cup extra-virgin olive oil

2 garlic cloves, minced

1 cup butterhead lettuce, torn into pieces

2 tablespoons fresh parsley, chopped

2 tablespoons fresh cilantro, chopped

1 teaspoon fresh basil

1 teaspoon fresh oregano

1 ½ cups cherry tomatoes, halved

3 ounces Kalamata olives, pitted and halved

Directions

In a large-sized saucepan, bring 4 ½ cups of the water and the red lentils to a boil.

Immediately turn the heat to a simmer and continue to cook your lentils for about 15 minutes or until tender. Drain and let it cool completely.

Transfer the lentils to a salad bowl; toss the lentils with the remaining ingredients until well combined.

Serve chilled or at room temperature. Bon appétit!

Roasted Asparagus and Avocado Salad

(Ready in about 20 minutes + chilling time | Servings 4)

Per serving : Calories: 378; Fat: 33.2g; Carbs: 18.6g; Protein: 7.8g

Ingredients

1 pound asparagus, trimmed, cut into bite-sized pieces

1 white onion, chopped

2 garlic cloves, minced

1 Roma tomato, sliced

1/4 cup olive oil

1/4 cup balsamic vinegar

1 tablespoon stone-ground mustard

2 tablespoons fresh parsley, chopped

1 tablespoon fresh cilantro, chopped

1 tablespoon fresh basil, chopped

Sea salt and ground black pepper, to taste

1 small avocado, pitted and diced

1/2 cup pine nuts, roughly chopped

Directions

Begin by preheating your oven to 420 degrees F.

Toss the asparagus with 1 tablespoon of the olive oil and arrange them on a parchment-lined roasting pan.

Bake for about 15 minutes, rotating the pan once or twice to promote even cooking. Let it cool completely and place in your salad bowl.

Toss the asparagus with the vegetables, olive oil, vinegar, mustard and herbs. Salt and pepper to taste.

Toss to combine and top with avocado and pine nuts. Bon appétit!

Creamed Green Bean Salad with Pine Nuts

(Ready in about 10 minutes + chilling time | Servings 5)

Per serving : Calories: 308; Fat: 26.2g; Carbs: 16.6g; Protein: 5.8g

Ingredients

1 ½ pounds green beans, trimmed

2 medium tomatoes, diced

2 bell peppers, seeded and diced

4 tablespoons shallots, chopped

1/2 cup pine nuts, roughly chopped

1/2 cup vegan mayonnaise

1 tablespoon deli mustard

2 tablespoons fresh basil, chopped

2 tablespoons fresh parsley, chopped

1/2 teaspoon red pepper flakes, crushed

Sea salt and freshly ground black pepper, to taste

Directions

Boil the green beans in a large saucepan of salted water until they are just tender or about 2 minutes.

Drain and let the beans cool completely; then, transfer them to a salad bowl. Toss the beans with the remaining ingredients.

Taste and adjust the seasonings. Bon appétit!

Cannellini Bean Soup with Kale

(Ready in about 25 minutes | Servings 5)

Per serving : Calories: 188; Fat: 4.7g; Carbs: 24.5g; Protein: 11.1g

Ingredients

1 tablespoon olive oil

1/2 teaspoon ginger, minced

1/2 teaspoon cumin seeds

1 red onion, chopped

1 carrot, trimmed and chopped

1 parsnip, trimmed and chopped

2 garlic cloves, minced

5 cups vegetable broth

12 ounces Cannellini beans, drained

2 cups kale, torn into pieces

Sea salt and ground black pepper, to taste

Directions

In a heavy-bottomed pot, heat the olive over medium-high heat. Now, sauté the ginger and cumin for 1 minute or so.

Now, add in the onion, carrot and parsnip; continue sautéing an additional 3 minutes or until the vegetables are just tender.

Add in the garlic and continue to sauté for 1 minute or until aromatic.

Then, pour in the vegetable broth and bring to a boil. Immediately reduce the heat to a simmer and let it cook for 10 minutes.

Fold in the Cannellini beans and kale; continue to simmer until the kale wilts and everything is thoroughly heated. Season with salt and pepper to taste.

Ladle into individual bowls and serve hot. Bon appétit!

. Hearty Cream of Mushroom Soup

(Ready in about 15 minutes | Servings 5)

Per serving : Calories: 308; Fat: 25.5g; Carbs: 11.8g; Protein: 11.6g

Ingredients

2 tablespoons soy butter

1 large shallot, chopped

20 ounces Cremini mushrooms, sliced

2 cloves garlic, minced

4 tablespoons flaxseed meal

5 cups vegetable broth

1 1/3 cups full-fat coconut milk

1 bay leaf

Sea salt and ground black pepper, to taste

Directions

In a stockpot, melt the vegan butter over medium-high heat. Once hot, cook the shallot for about 3 minutes until tender and fragrant.

Add in the mushrooms and garlic and continue cooking until the mushrooms have softened. Add in the flaxseed meal and continue to cook for 1 minute or so.

Add in the remaining ingredients. Let it simmer, covered and continue to cook for 5 to 6 minutes more until your soup has thickened slightly.

Bon appétit!

Authentic Italian Panzanella Salad

(Ready in about 35 minutes | Servings 3)

Per serving : Calories: 334; Fat: 20.4g; Carbs: 33.3g; Protein: 8.3g

Ingredients

3 cups artisan bread, broken into 1-inch cubes

3/4 pound asparagus, trimmed and cut into bite-sized pieces

4 tablespoons extra-virgin olive oil

1 red onion, chopped

2 tablespoons fresh lime juice

1 teaspoon deli mustard

2 medium heirloom tomatoes, diced

2 cups arugula

2 cups baby spinach

2 Italian peppers, seeded and sliced

Sea salt and ground black pepper, to taste

Directions

Arrange the bread cubes on a parchment-lined baking sheet. Bake in the preheated oven at 310 degrees F for about 20 minutes, rotating the baking sheet twice during the baking time; reserve.

Turn the oven to 420 degrees F and toss the asparagus with 1 tablespoon of olive oil. Roast the asparagus for about 15 minutes or until crisp-tender.

Toss the remaining ingredients in a salad bowl; top with the roasted asparagus and toasted bread.

Bon appétit!

Quinoa and Black Bean Salad

(Ready in about 15 minutes + chilling time | Servings 4)

Per serving : Calories: 433; Fat: 17.3g; Carbs: 57g; Protein: 15.1g

Ingredients

2 cups water

1 cup quinoa, rinsed

16 ounces canned black beans, drained

2 Roma tomatoes, sliced

1 red onion, thinly sliced

1 cucumber, seeded and chopped

2 cloves garlic, pressed or minced

2 Italian peppers, seeded and sliced

2 tablespoons fresh parsley, chopped

2 tablespoons fresh cilantro, chopped

1/4 cup olive oil

1 lemon, freshly squeezed

1 tablespoon apple cider vinegar

1/2 teaspoon dried dill weed

1/2 teaspoon dried oregano

Sea salt and ground black pepper, to tast e

Directions

Place the water and quinoa in a saucepan and bring it to a rolling boil. Immediately turn the heat to a simmer.

Let it simmer for about 13 minutes until the quinoa has absorbed all of the water; fluff the quinoa with a fork and let it cool completely. Then, transfer the quinoa to a salad bowl.

Add the remaining ingredients to the salad bowl and toss to combine well. Bon appétit!

Rich Bulgur Salad with Herbs

(Ready in about 20 minutes + chilling time | Servings 4)

Per serving : Calories: 408; Fat: 18.3g; Carbs: 51.8g; Protein: 13.1g

Ingredients

2 cups water

1 cup bulgur

12 ounces canned chickpeas, drained

1 Persian cucumber, thinly sliced

2 bell peppers, seeded and thinly sliced

1 jalapeno pepper, seeded and thinly sliced

2 Roma tomatoes, sliced

1 onion, thinly sliced

2 tablespoons fresh basil, chopped

2 tablespoons fresh parsley, chopped

2 tablespoons fresh mint, chopped

2 tablespoons fresh chives, chopped

4 tablespoons olive oil

1 tablespoon balsamic vinegar

1 tablespoon lemon juice

1 teaspoon fresh garlic, pressed

Sea salt and freshly ground black pepper, to taste

2 tablespoons nutritional yeast

1/2 cup Kalamata olives, sliced

Directions

In a saucepan, bring the water and bulgur to a boil. Immediately turn the heat to a simmer and let it cook for about 20 minutes or until the bulgur is tender and water is almost absorbed. Fluff with a fork and spread on a large tray to let cool.

Place the bulgur in a salad bowl followed by the chickpeas, cucumber, peppers, tomatoes, onion, basil, parsley, mint and chives.

In a small mixing dish, whisk the olive oil, balsamic vinegar, lemon juice, garlic, salt and black pepper. Dress the salad and toss to combine.

Sprinkle nutritional yeast over the top, garnish with olives and serve at room temperature. Bon appétit!

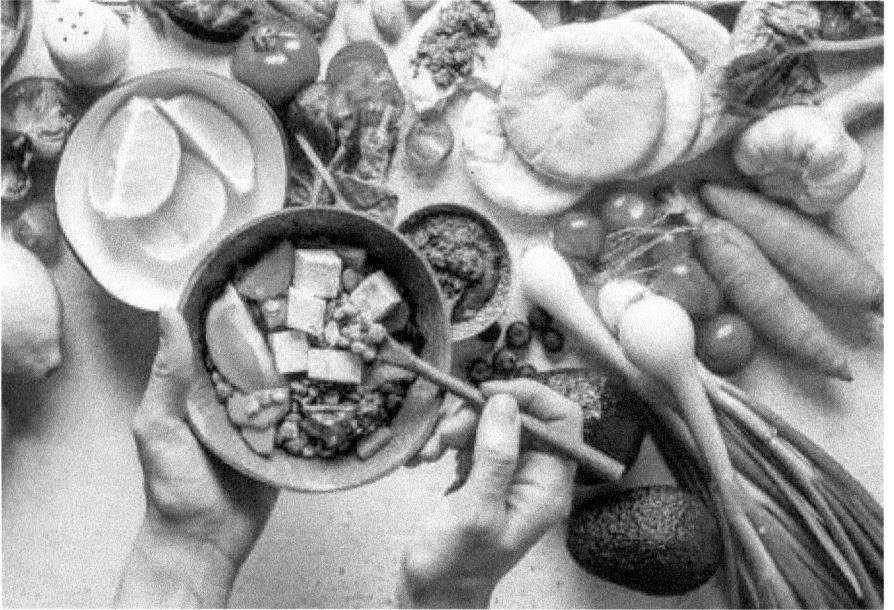

Classic Roasted Pepper Salad

(Ready in about 15 minutes + chilling time | Servings 3)

Per serving : Calories: 178; Fat: 14.4g; Carbs: 11.8g; Protein: 2.4g

Ingredients

6 bell peppers

3 tablespoons extra-virgin olive oil

3 teaspoons red wine vinegar

3 garlic cloves, finely chopped

2 tablespoons fresh parsley, chopped

Sea salt and freshly cracked black pepper, to taste

1/2 teaspoon red pepper flakes

6 tablespoons pine nuts, roughly chopped

Directions

Broil the peppers on a parchment-lined baking sheet for about 10 minutes, rotating the pan halfway through the cooking time, until they are charred on all sides.

Then, cover the peppers with a plastic wrap to steam. Discard the skin, seeds and cores.

Slice the peppers into strips and toss them with the remaining ingredients. Place in your refrigerator until ready to serve. Bon appétit!

Hearty Winter Quinoa Soup

(Ready in about 25 minutes | Servings 4)

Per serving : Calories: 328; Fat: 11.1g; Carbs: 44.1g; Protein: 13.3g

Ingredients

2 tablespoons olive oil

1 onion, chopped

2 carrots, peeled and chopped

1 parsnip, chopped

1 celery stalk, chopped

1 cup yellow squash, chopped

4 garlic cloves, pressed or minced

4 cups roasted vegetable broth

2 medium tomatoes, crushed

1 cup quinoa

Sea salt and ground black pepper, to taste

1 bay laurel

2 cup Swiss chard, tough ribs removed and torn into pieces

2 tablespoons Italian parsley, chopped

Directions

In a heavy-bottomed pot, heat the olive over medium-high heat. Now, sauté the onion, carrot, parsnip, celery and yellow squash for about 3 minutes or until the vegetables are just tender.

Add in the garlic and continue to sauté for 1 minute or until aromatic.

Then, stir in the vegetable broth, tomatoes, quinoa, salt, pepper and bay laurel; bring to a boil. Immediately reduce the heat to a simmer and let it cook for 13 minutes.

Fold in the Swiss chard; continue to simmer until the chard wilts.

Ladle into individual bowls and serve garnished with the fresh parsley. Bon appétit!

Green Lentil Salad

(Ready in about 20 minutes + chilling time | Servings 5)

Per serving : Calories: 349; Fat: 15.1g; Carbs: 40.9g; Protein: 15.4g

Ingredients

1 ½ cups green lentils, rinsed

2 cups arugula

2 cups Romaine lettuce, torn into pieces

1 cup baby spinach

1/4 cup fresh basil, chopped

1/2 cup shallots, chopped

2 garlic cloves, finely chopped

1/4 cup oil-packed sun-dried tomatoes, rinsed and chopped

5 tablespoons extra-virgin olive oil

3 tablespoons fresh lemon juice

Sea salt and ground black pepper, to taste

Directions

In a large-sized saucepan, bring 4 ½ cups of the water and red lentils to a boil.

Immediately turn the heat to a simmer and continue to cook your lentils for a further 15 to 17 minutes or until they've softened but not mushy. Drain and let it cool completely.

Transfer the lentils to a salad bowl; toss the lentils with the remaining ingredients until well combined.

Serve chilled or at room temperature. Bon appétit!

. Acorn Squash, Chickpea and Couscous Soup

(Ready in about 20 minutes | Servings 4)

Per serving : Calories: 378; Fat: 11g; Carbs: 60.1g; Protein: 10.9g

Ingredients

2 tablespoons olive oil

1 shallot, chopped

1 carrot, trimmed and chopped

2 cups acorn squash, chopped

1 stalk celery, chopped

1 teaspoon garlic, finely chopped

1 teaspoon dried rosemary, chopped

1 teaspoon dried thyme, chopped

2 cups cream of onion soup

2 cups water

1 cup dry couscous

Sea salt and ground black pepper, to taste

1/2 teaspoon red pepper flakes

6 ounces canned chickpeas, drained

2 tablespoons fresh lemon juice

Directions

In a heavy-bottomed pot, heat the olive over medium-high heat. Now, sauté the shallot, carrot, acorn squash and celery for about 3 minutes or until the vegetables are just tender.

Add in the garlic, rosemary and thyme and continue to sauté for 1 minute or until aromatic.

Then, stir in the soup, water, couscous, salt, black pepper and red pepper flakes; bring to a boil. Immediately reduce the heat to a simmer and let it cook for 12 minutes.

Fold in the canned chickpeas; continue to simmer until heated through or about 5 minutes more.

Ladle into individual bowls and drizzle with the lemon juice over the top. Bon appétit!

. Cabbage Soup with Garlic Crostini

(Ready in about 1 hour | Servings 4)

Per serving : Calories: 408; Fat: 23.1g; Carbs: 37.6g; Protein: 11.8g

Ingredients

Soup:

2 tablespoons olive oil

1 medium leek, chopped

1 cup turnip, chopped

1 parsnip, chopped

1 carrot, chopped

2 cups cabbage, shredded

2 garlic cloves, finely chopped

4 cups vegetable broth

2 bay leaves

Sea salt and ground black pepper, to taste

1/4 teaspoon cumin seeds

1/2 teaspoon mustard seeds

1 teaspoon dried basil

2 tomatoes, pureed

Crostini:

8 slices of baguette

2 heads garlic

4 tablespoons extra-virgin olive oil

Directions

In a soup pot, heat 2 tablespoons of the olive over medium-high heat. Now, sauté the leek, turnip, parsnip and carrot for about 4 minutes or until the vegetables are crisp-tender.

Add in the garlic and cabbage and continue to sauté for 1 minute or until aromatic.

Then, stir in the vegetable broth, bay leaves, salt, black pepper, cumin seeds, mustard seeds, dried basil and pureed tomatoes; bring to a boil. Immediately reduce the heat to a simmer and let it cook for about 20 minutes.

Meanwhile, preheat your oven to 375 degrees F. Now, roast the garlic and baguette slices for about 15 minutes. Remove the crostini from the oven.

Continue baking the garlic for 45 minutes more or until very tender. Allow the garlic to cool.

Now, cut each head of the garlic using a sharp serrated knife in order to separate all the cloves.

Squeeze the roasted garlic cloves out of their skins. Mash the garlic pulp with 4 tablespoons of the extra-virgin olive oil.

Spread the roasted garlic mixture evenly on the tops of the crostini. Serve with the warm soup. Bon appétit!

Cream of Green Bean Soup

(Ready in about 35 minutes | Servings 4)

Per serving : Calories: 410; Fat: 19.6g; Carbs: 50.6g; Protein: 13.3g

Ingredients

1 tablespoon sesame oil

1 onion, chopped

1 green pepper, seeded and chopped

2 russet potatoes, peeled and diced

2 garlic cloves, chopped

4 cups vegetable broth

1 pound green beans, trimmed

Sea salt and ground black pepper, to season

1 cup full-fat coconut milk

Directions

In a heavy-bottomed pot, heat the sesame over medium-high heat. Now, sauté the onion, peppers and potatoes for about 5 minutes, stirring periodically.

Add in the garlic and continue sautéing for 1 minute or until fragrant.

Then, stir in the vegetable broth, green beans, salt and black pepper; bring to a boil. Immediately reduce the heat to a simmer and let it cook for 20 minutes.

Puree the green bean mixture using an immersion blender until creamy and uniform.

Return the pureed mixture to the pot. Fold in the coconut milk and continue to simmer until heated through or about 5 minutes longer.

Ladle into individual bowls and serve hot. Bon appétit!

Traditional French Onion Soup

(Ready in about 1 hour 30 minutes | Servings 4)

Per serving : Calories: 129; Fat: 8.6g; Carbs: 7.4g; Protein: 6.3g

Ingredients

2 tablespoons olive oil

2 large yellow onions, thinly sliced

2 thyme sprigs, chopped

2 rosemary sprigs, chopped

2 teaspoons balsamic vinegar

4 cups vegetable stock

Sea salt and ground black pepper, to taste

Directions

In a or Dutch oven, heat the olive oil over a moderate heat. Now, cook the onions with thyme, rosemary and 1 teaspoon of the sea salt for about 2 minutes.

Now, turn the heat to medium-low and continue cooking until the onions caramelize or about 50 minutes.

Add in the balsamic vinegar and continue to cook for a further 15 more. Add in the stock, salt and black pepper and continue simmering for 20 to 25 minutes.

Serve with toasted bread and enjoy!

. Roasted Carrot Soup

(Ready in about 50 minutes | Servings 4)

Per serving : Calories: 264; Fat: 18.6g; Carbs: 20.1g; Protein: 7.4g

Ingredients

1 ½ pounds carrots

4 tablespoons olive oil

1 yellow onion, chopped

2 cloves garlic, minced

1/3 teaspoon ground cumin

Sea salt and white pepper, to taste

1/2 teaspoon turmeric powder

4 cups vegetable stock

2 teaspoons lemon juice

2 tablespoons fresh cilantro, roughly chopped

Directions

Start by preheating your oven to 400 degrees F. Place the carrots on a large parchment-lined baking sheet; toss the carrots with 2 tablespoons of the olive oil.

Roast the carrots for about 35 minutes or until they've softened.

In a heavy-bottomed pot, heat the remaining 2 tablespoons of the olive oil. Now, sauté the onion and garlic for about 3 minutes or until aromatic.

Add in the cumin, salt, pepper, turmeric, vegetable stock and roasted carrots. Continue to simmer for 12 minutes more.

Puree your soup with an immersion blender. Drizzle lemon juice over your soup and serve garnished with fresh cilantro leaves. Bon appétit!

Italian Penne Pasta Salad

(Ready in about 15 minutes + chilling time | Servings 3)

Per serving : Calories: 614; Fat: 18.1g; Carbs: 101g; Protein: 15.4g

Ingredients

9 ounces penne pasta

9 ounces canned Cannellini bean, drained

1 small onion, thinly sliced

1/3 cup Niçoise olives, pitted and sliced

2 Italian peppers, sliced

1 cup cherry tomatoes, halved

3 cups arugula

Dressing:

3 tablespoons extra-virgin olive oil

1 teaspoon lemon zest

1 teaspoon garlic, minced

3 tablespoons balsamic vinegar

1 teaspoon Italian herb mix

Sea salt and ground black pepper, to taste

Directions

Cook the penne pasta according to the package directions. Drain and rinse the pasta. Let it cool completely and then, transfer it to a salad bowl.

Then, add the beans, onion, olives, peppers, tomatoes and arugula to the salad bowl.

Mix all the dressing ingredients until everything is well incorporated. Dress your salad and serve well-chilled. Bon appétit!

Indian Chana Chaat Salad

(Ready in about 45 minutes + chilling time | Servings 4)

Per serving : Calories: 604; Fat: 23.1g; Carbs: 80g; Protein: 25.3g

Ingredients

1 pound dry chickpeas, soaked overnight

2 San Marzano tomatoes, diced

1 Persian cucumber, sliced

1 onion, chopped

1 bell pepper, seeded and thinly sliced

1 green chili, seeded and thinly sliced

2 handfuls baby spinach

1/2 teaspoon Kashmiri chili powder

4 curry leaves, chopped

1 tablespoon chaat masala

2 tablespoons fresh lemon juice, or to taste

4 tablespoons olive oil

1 teaspoon agave syrup

1/2 teaspoon mustard seeds

1/2 teaspoon coriander seeds

2 tablespoons sesame seeds, lightly toasted

2 tablespoons fresh cilantro, roughly chopped

Directions

Drain the chickpeas and transfer them to a large saucepan. Cover the chickpeas with water by 2 inches and bring it to a boil.

Immediately turn the heat to a simmer and continue to cook for approximately 40 minutes.

Toss the chickpeas with the tomatoes, cucumber, onion, peppers, spinach, chili powder, curry leaves and chaat masala.

In a small mixing dish, thoroughly combine the lemon juice, olive oil, agave syrup, mustard seeds and coriander seeds.

Garnish with sesame seeds and fresh cilantro. Bon appétit!

Thai-Style Tempeh and Noodle Salad

(Ready in about 45 minutes | Servings 3)

Per serving : Calories: 494; Fat: 14.5g; Carbs: 75g; Protein: 18.7g

Ingredients

6 ounces tempeh

4 tablespoons rice vinegar

4 tablespoons soy sauce

2 garlic cloves, minced

1 small-sized lime, freshly juiced

5 ounces rice noodles

1 carrot, julienned

1 shallot, chopped

3 handfuls Chinese cabbage, thinly sliced

3 handfuls kale, torn into pieces

1 bell pepper, seeded and thinly sliced

1 bird's eye chili, minced

1/4 cup peanut butter

2 tablespoons agave syrup

Directions

Place the tempeh, 2 tablespoons of the rice vinegar, soy sauce, garlic and lime juice in a ceramic dish; let it marinate for about 40 minutes.

Meanwhile, cook the rice noodles according to the package directions. Drain your noodles and transfer them to a salad bowl.

Add the carrot, shallot, cabbage, kale and peppers to the salad bowl. Add in the peanut butter, the remaining 2 tablespoons of the rice vinegar and agave syrup and toss to combine well.

Top with the marinated tempeh and serve immediately. Enjoy!

Classic Cream of Broccoli Soup

(Ready in about 35 minutes | Servings 4)

Per serving : Calories: 334; Fat: 24.5g; Carbs: 22.5g; Protein: 10.2g

Ingredients

2 tablespoons olive oil

1 pound broccoli florets

1 onion, chopped

1 celery rib, chopped

1 parsnip, chopped

1 teaspoon garlic, chopped

3 cups vegetable broth

1/2 teaspoon dried dill

1/2 teaspoon dried oregano

Sea salt and ground black pepper, to taste

2 tablespoons flaxseed meal

1 cup full-fat coconut milk

Directions

In a heavy-bottomed pot, heat the olive oil over medium-high heat. Now, sauté the broccoli onion, celery and parsnip for about 5 minutes, stirring periodically.

Add in the garlic and continue sautéing for 1 minute or until fragrant.

Then, stir in the vegetable broth, dill, oregano, salt and black pepper; bring to a boil. Immediately reduce the heat to a simmer and let it cook for about 20 minutes.

Puree the soup using an immersion blender until creamy and uniform.

Return the pureed mixture to the pot. Fold in the flaxseed meal and coconut milk; continue to simmer until heated through or about 5 minutes.

Ladle into four serving bowls and enjoy!

Moroccan Lentil and Raisin Salad

(Ready in about 20 minutes + chilling time | Servings 4)

Per serving : Calories: 418; Fat: 15g; Carbs: 62.9g; Protein: 12.4g

Ingredients

1 cup red lentils, rinsed

1 large carrot, julienned

1 Persian cucumber, thinly sliced

1 sweet onion, chopped

1/2 cup golden raisins

1/4 cup fresh mint, snipped

1/4 cup fresh basil, snipped

1/4 cup extra-virgin olive oil

1/4 cup lemon juice, freshly squeezed

1 teaspoon grated lemon peel

1/2 teaspoon fresh ginger root, peeled and minced

1/2 teaspoon granulated garlic

1 teaspoon ground allspice

Sea salt and ground black pepper, to taste

Directions

In a large-sized saucepan, bring 3 cups of the water and 1 cup of the lentils to a boil.

Immediately turn the heat to a simmer and continue to cook your lentils for a further 15 to 17 minutes or until they've softened but are not mushy yet. Drain and let it cool completely.

Transfer the lentils to a salad bowl; add in the carrot, cucumber and sweet onion. Then, add the raisins, mint and basil to your salad.

In a small mixing dish, whisk the olive oil, lemon juice, lemon peel, ginger, granulated garlic, allspice, salt and black pepper.

Dress your salad and serve well-chilled. Bon appétit!

Asparagus and Chickpea Salad

(Ready in about 10 minutes + chilling time | Servings 5)

Per serving : Calories: 198; Fat: 12.9g; Carbs: 17.5g; Protein: 5.5g

Ingredients

1 ¼ pounds asparagus, trimmed and cut into bite-sized pieces

5 ounces canned chickpeas, drained and rinsed

1 chipotle pepper, seeded and chopped

1 Italian pepper, seeded and chopped

1/4 cup fresh basil leaves, chopped

1/4 cup fresh parsley leaves, chopped

2 tablespoons fresh mint leaves

2 tablespoons fresh chives, chopped

1 teaspoon garlic, minced

1/4 cup extra-virgin olive oil

1 tablespoon balsamic vinegar

1 tablespoon fresh lime juice

2 tablespoons soy sauce

1/4 teaspoon ground allspice

1/4 teaspoon ground cumin

Sea salt and freshly cracked peppercorns, to tast e

Directions

Bring a large pot of salted water with the asparagus to a boil; let it cook for 2 minutes; drain and rinse.

Transfer the asparagus to a salad bowl.

Toss the asparagus with the chickpeas, peppers, herbs, garlic, olive oil, vinegar, lime juice, soy sauce and spices.

Toss to combine and serve immediately. Bon appétit!

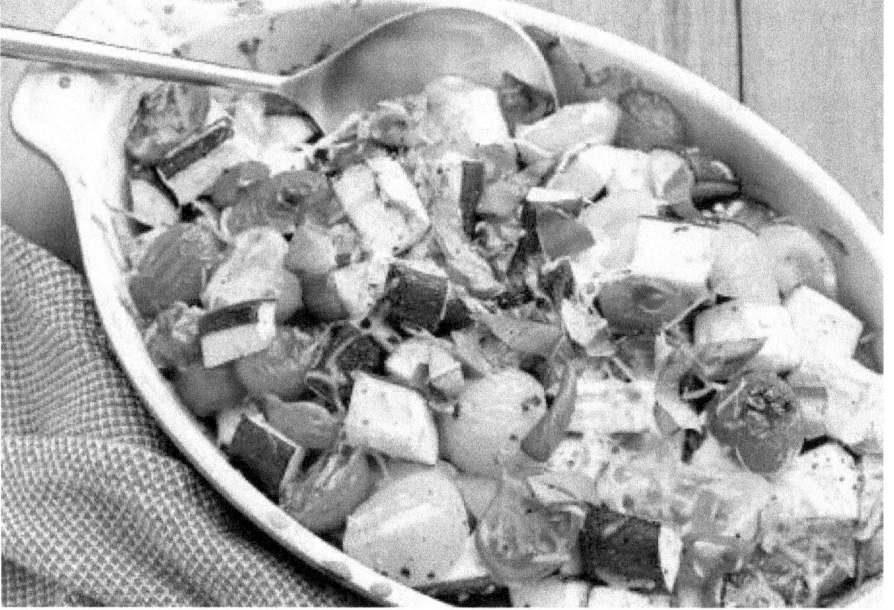

Old-Fashioned Green Bean Salad

(Ready in about 10 minutes + chilling time | Servings 4)

Per serving : Calories: 240; Fat: 14.1g; Carbs: 29g; Protein: 4.4g

Ingredients

1 ½ pounds green beans, trimmed

1/2 cup scallions, chopped

1 teaspoon garlic, minced

1 Persian cucumber, sliced

2 cups grape tomatoes, halved

1/4 cup olive oil

1 teaspoon deli mustard

2 tablespoons tamari sauce

2 tablespoons lemon juice

1 tablespoon apple cider vinegar

1/4 teaspoon cumin powder

1/2 teaspoon dried thyme

Sea salt and ground black pepper, to taste

Directions

Boil the green beans in a large saucepan of salted water until they are just tender or about 2 minutes.

Drain and let the beans cool completely; then, transfer them to a salad bowl. Toss the beans with the remaining ingredients.

Bon appétit!

Winter Bean Soup

(Ready in about 25 minutes | Servings 4)

Per serving : Calories: 234; Fat: 5.5g; Carbs: 32.3g; Protein: 14.4g

Ingredients

1 tablespoon olive oil

2 tablespoons shallots, chopped

1 carrot, chopped

1 parsnip, chopped

1 celery stalk, chopped

1 teaspoon fresh garlic, minced

4 cups vegetable broth

2 bay leaves

1 rosemary sprig, chopped

16 ounces canned navy beans

Flaky sea salt and ground black pepper, to taste

Directions

In a heavy-bottomed pot, heat the olive over medium-high heat. Now, sauté the shallots, carrot, parsnip and celery for approximately 3 minutes or until the vegetables are just tender.

Add in the garlic and continue to sauté for 1 minute or until aromatic.

Then, add in the vegetable broth, bay leaves and rosemary and bring to a boil. Immediately reduce the heat to a simmer and let it cook for 10 minutes.

Fold in the navy beans and continue to simmer for about 5 minutes longer until everything is thoroughly heated. Season with salt and black pepper to taste.

Ladle into individual bowls, discard the bay leaves and serve hot. Bon appétit!

Italian-Style Cremini Mushrooms Soup

(Ready in about 15 minutes | Servings 3)

Per serving : Calories: 154; Fat: 12.3g; Carbs: 9.6g; Protein: 4.4g

Ingredients

3 tablespoons vegan butter

1 white onion, chopped

1 red bell pepper, chopped

1/2 teaspoon garlic, pressed

3 cups Cremini mushrooms, chopped

2 tablespoons almond flour

3 cups water

1 teaspoon Italian herb mix

Sea salt and ground black pepper, to taste

1 heaping tablespoon fresh chives, roughly chopped

Directions

In a stockpot, melt the vegan butter over medium-high heat. Once hot, sauté the onion and pepper for about 3 minutes until they have softened.

Add in the garlic and Cremini mushrooms and continue sautéing until the mushrooms have softened. Sprinkle almond meal over the mushrooms and continue to cook for 1 minute or so.

Add in the remaining ingredients. Let it simmer, covered and continue to cook for 5 to 6 minutes more until the liquid has thickened slightly.

Ladle into three soup bowls and garnish with fresh chives. Bon appétit!

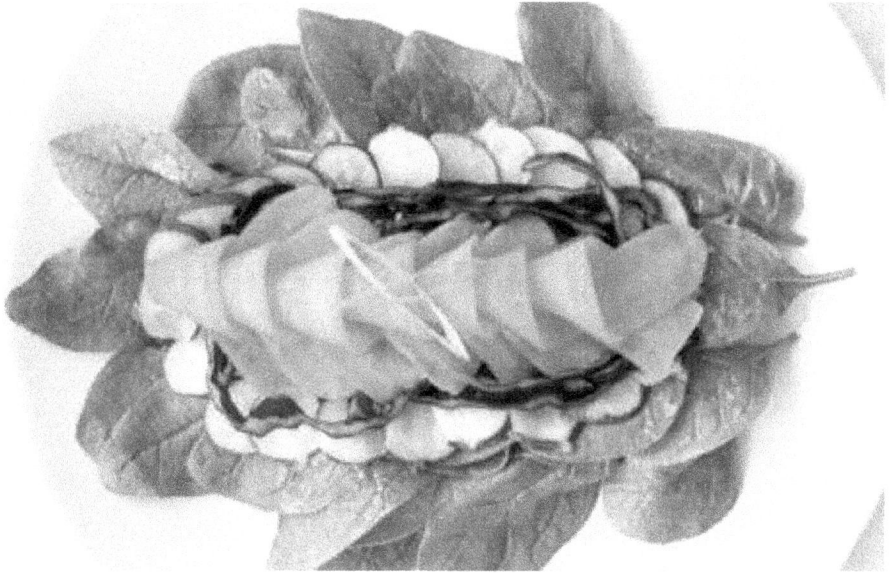

Creamed Potato Soup with Herbs

(Ready in about 40 minutes | Servings 4)

Per serving : Calories: 400; Fat: 9g; Carbs: 68.7g; Protein: 13.4g

Ingredients

2 tablespoons olive oil

1 onion, chopped

1 celery stalk, chopped

4 large potatoes, peeled and chopped

2 garlic cloves, minced

1 teaspoon fresh basil, chopped

1 teaspoon fresh parsley, chopped

1 teaspoon fresh rosemary, chopped

1 bay laurel

1 teaspoon ground allspice

4 cups vegetable stock

Salt and fresh ground black pepper, to taste

2 tablespoons fresh chives chopped

Directions

In a heavy-bottomed pot, heat the olive oil over medium-high heat. Once hot, sauté the onion, celery and potatoes for about 5 minutes, stirring periodically.

Add in the garlic, basil, parsley, rosemary, bay laurel and allspice and continue sautéing for 1 minute or until fragrant.

Now, add in the vegetable stock, salt and black pepper and bring to a rapid boil. Immediately reduce the heat to a simmer and let it cook for about 30 minutes.

Puree the soup using an immersion blender until creamy and uniform.

Reheat your soup and serve with fresh chives. Bon appétit!

Quinoa and Avocado Salad

(Ready in about 15 minutes + chilling time | Servings 4)

Per serving : Calories: 399; Fat: 24.3g; Carbs: 38.5g; Protein: 8.4g

Ingredients

1 cup quinoa, rinsed

1 onion, chopped

1 tomato, diced

2 roasted peppers, cut into strips

2 tablespoons parsley, chopped

2 tablespoons basil, chopped

1/4 cup extra-virgin olive oil

2 tablespoons red wine vinegar

2 tablespoons lemon juice

1/4 teaspoon cayenne pepper

Sea salt and freshly ground black pepper, to season

1 avocado, peeled, pitted and sliced

1 tablespoon sesame seeds, toasted

Directions

Place the water and quinoa in a saucepan and bring it to a rolling boil. Immediately turn the heat to a simmer.

Let it simmer for about 13 minutes until the quinoa has absorbed all of the water; fluff the quinoa with a fork and let it cool completely. Then, transfer the quinoa to a salad bowl.

Add the onion, tomato, roasted peppers, parsley and basil to the salad bowl. In another small bowl, whisk the olive oil, vinegar, lemon juice, cayenne pepper, salt and black pepper.

Dress your salad and toss to combine well. Top with avocado slices and garnish with toasted sesame seeds.

Bon appétit!

Tabbouleh Salad with Tofu

(Ready in about 20 minutes + chilling time | Servings 4)

Per serving : Calories: 379; Fat: 18.3g; Carbs: 40.7g; Protein: 19.9g

Ingredients

1 cup bulgur wheat

2 San Marzano tomatoes, sliced

1 Persian cucumber, thinly sliced

2 tablespoons basil, chopped

2 tablespoons parsley, chopped

4 scallions, chopped

2 cups arugula

2 cups baby spinach, torn into pieces

4 tablespoons tahini

4 tablespoons lemon juice

1 tablespoon soy sauce

1 teaspoon fresh garlic, pressed

Sea salt and ground black pepper, to taste

12 ounces smoked tofu, cubed

Directions

In a saucepan, bring 2 cups of water and the bulgur to a boil. Immediately turn the heat to a simmer and let it cook for about 20 minutes or until the bulgur is tender and the water is almost absorbed. Fluff with a fork and spread on a large tray to let cool.

Place the bulgur in a salad bowl followed by the tomatoes, cucumber, basil, parsley, scallions, arugula and spinach.

In a small mixing dish, whisk the tahini, lemon juice, soy sauce, garlic, salt and black pepper. Dress the salad and toss to combine.

Top your salad with the smoked tofu and serve at room temperature. Bon appétit!

Garden Pasta Salad

(Ready in about 10 minutes + chilling time | Servings 4)

Per serving : Calories: 479; Fat: 15g; Carbs: 71.1g; Protein: 14.9g

Ingredients

12 ounces rotini pasta

1 small onion, thinly sliced

1 cup cherry tomatoes, halved

1 bell pepper, chopped

1 jalapeno pepper, chopped

1 tablespoon capers, drained

2 cups Iceberg lettuce, torn into pieces

2 tablespoons fresh parsley, chopped

2 tablespoons fresh cilantro, chopped

2 tablespoons fresh basil, chopped

1/4 cup olive oil

2 tablespoons apple cider vinegar

1 teaspoon garlic, pressed

Kosher salt and ground black pepper, to taste

2 tablespoons nutritional yeast

2 tablespoons pine nuts, toasted and choppe d

Directions

Cook the pasta according to the package directions. Drain and rinse the pasta. Let it cool completely and then, transfer it to a salad bowl.

Then, add in the onion, tomatoes, peppers, capers, lettuce, parsley, cilantro and basil to the salad bowl.

Whisk the olive oil, vinegar, garlic, salt, black pepper and nutritional yeast. Dress your salad and top with toasted pine nuts. Bon appétit!

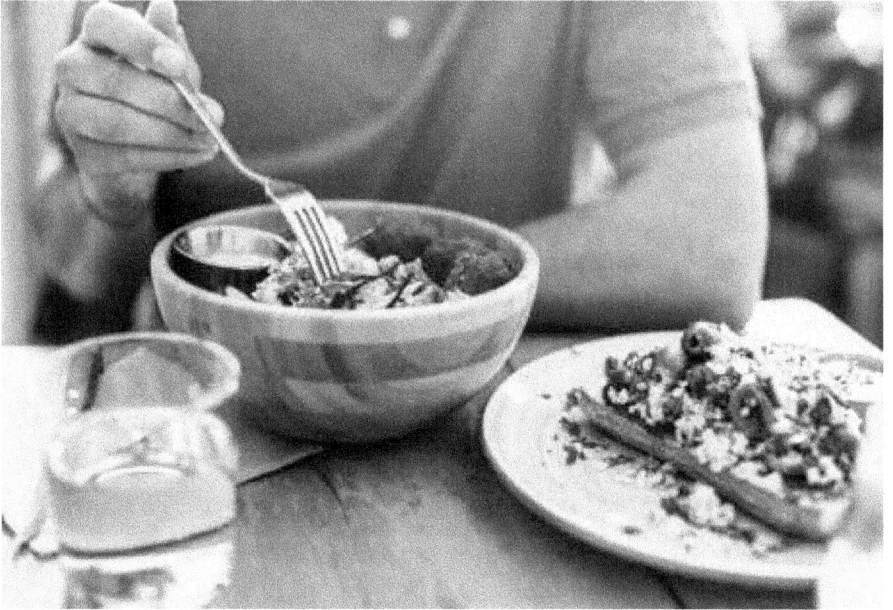

Traditional Ukrainian Borscht

(Ready in about 40 minutes | Servings 4)

Per serving : Calories: 367; Fat: 9.3g; Carbs: 62.7g; Protein: 12.1g

Ingredients

2 tablespoons sesame oil

1 red onion, chopped

2 carrots, trimmed and sliced

2 large beets, peeled and sliced

2 large potatoes, peeled and diced

4 cups vegetable stock

2 garlic cloves, minced

1/2 teaspoon caraway seeds

1/2 teaspoon celery seeds

1/2 teaspoon fennel seeds

1 pound red cabbage, shredded

1/2 teaspoon mixed peppercorns, freshly cracked

Kosher salt, to taste

2 bay leaves

2 tablespoons wine vinegar

Directions

In a Dutch oven, heat the sesame oil over a moderate flame. Once hot, sauté the onions until tender and translucent, about 6 minutes.

Add in the carrots, beets and potatoes and continue to sauté an additional 10 minutes, adding the vegetable stock periodically.

Next, stir in the garlic, caraway seeds, celery seeds, fennel seeds and continue sautéing for another 30 seconds.

Add in the cabbage, mixed peppercorns, salt and bay leaves. Add in the remaining stock and bring to boil.

Immediately turn the heat to a simmer and continue to cook for 20 to 23 minutes longer until the vegetables have softened.

Ladle into individual bowls and drizzle wine vinegar over it. Serve and enjoy!

Beluga Lentil Salad

(Ready in about 20 minutes + chilling time | Servings 4)

Per serving : Calories: 338; Fat: 16.3g; Carbs: 37.2g; Protein: 13g

Ingredients

1 cup Beluga lentils, rinsed

1 Persian cucumber, sliced

1 large-sized tomatoes, sliced

1 red onion, chopped

1 bell pepper, sliced

1/4 cup fresh basil, chopped

1/4 cup fresh Italian parsley, chopped

2 ounces green olives, pitted and sliced

1/4 cup olive oil

4 tablespoons lemon juice

1 teaspoon deli mustard

1/2 teaspoon garlic, minced

1/2 teaspoon red pepper flakes, crushed

Sea salt and ground black pepper, to taste

Directions

In a large-sized saucepan, bring 3 cups of the water and 1 cup of the lentils to a boil.

Immediately turn the heat to a simmer and continue to cook your lentils for a further 15 to 17 minutes or until they've softened but not mushy. Drain and let it cool completely.

Transfer the lentils to a salad bowl; add in the cucumber, tomatoes, onion, pepper, basil, parsley and olives.

In a small mixing dish, whisk the olive oil, lemon juice, mustard, garlic, red pepper, salt and black pepper.

Dress the salad, toss to combine and serve well-chilled. Bon appétit!

Indian-Style Naan Salad

(Ready in about 10 minutes | Servings 3)

Per serving : Calories: 328; Fat: 17.3g; Carbs: 36.6g; Protein: 6.9g

Ingredients

3 tablespoons sesame oil

1 teaspoon ginger, peeled and minced

1/2 teaspoon cumin seeds

1/2 teaspoon mustard seeds

1/2 teaspoon mixed peppercorns

1 tablespoon curry leaves

3 naan breads, broken into bite-sized pieces

1 shallot, chopped

2 tomatoes, chopped

Himalayan salt, to taste

1 tablespoon soy sauce

Directions

Heat 2 tablespoons of the sesame oil in a nonstick skillet over a moderately high heat.

Sauté the ginger, cumin seeds, mustard seeds, mixed peppercorns and curry leaves for 1 minute or so, until fragrant.

Stir in the naan breads and continue to cook, stirring periodically, until golden-brown and well coated with the spices.

Place the shallot and tomatoes in a salad bowl; toss them with the salt, soy sauce and the remaining 1 tablespoon of the sesame oil.

Place the toasted naan on the top of your salad and serve at room temperature. Enjoy!

Greek-Style Roasted Pepper Salad

(Ready in about 10 minutes | Servings 2)

Per serving : Calories: 185; Fat: 11.5g; Carbs: 20.6g; Protein: 3.7g

Ingredients

2 red bell peppers

2 yellow bell peppers

2 garlic cloves, pressed

4 teaspoons extra-virgin olive oil

1 tablespoon capers, rinsed and drained

2 tablespoons red wine vinegar

Seas salt and ground pepper, to taste

1 teaspoon fresh dill weed, chopped

1 teaspoon fresh oregano, chopped

1/4 cup Kalamata olives, pitted and sliced

Directions

Broil the peppers on a parchment-lined baking sheet for about 10 minutes, rotating the pan halfway through the cooking time, until they are charred on all sides.

Then, cover the peppers with a plastic wrap to steam. Discard the skin, seeds and cores.

Slice the peppers into strips and place them in a salad bowl. Add in the remaining ingredients and toss to combine well.

Place in your refrigerator until ready to serve. Bon appétit!

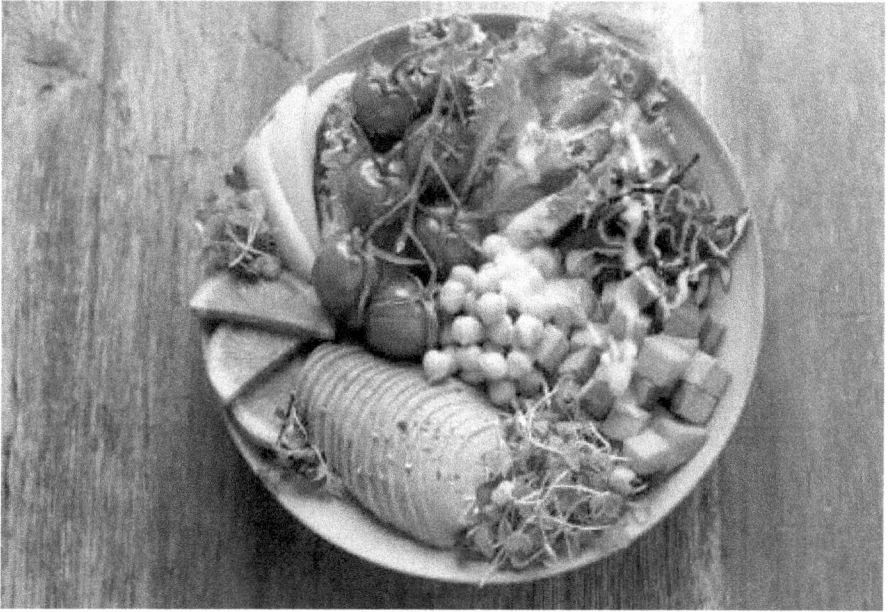

Kidney Bean and Potato Soup

(Ready in about 30 minutes | Servings 4)

Per serving : Calories: 266; Fat: 7.7g; Carbs: 41.3g; Protein: 9.3g

Ingredients

2 tablespoons olive oil

1 onion, chopped

1 pound potatoes, peeled and diced

1 medium celery stalks, chopped

2 garlic cloves, minced

1 teaspoon paprika

4 cups water

2 tablespoons vegan bouillon powder

16 ounces canned kidney beans, drained

2 cups baby spinach

Sea salt and ground black pepper, to taste

Directions

In a heavy-bottomed pot, heat the olive over medium-high heat. Now, sauté the onion, potatoes and celery for approximately 5 minutes or until the onion is translucent and tender.

Add in the garlic and continue to sauté for 1 minute or until aromatic.

Then, add in the paprika, water and vegan bouillon powder and bring to a boil. Immediately reduce the heat to a simmer and let it cook for 15 minutes.

Fold in the navy beans and spinach; continue to simmer for about 5 minutes until everything is thoroughly heated. Season with salt and black pepper to taste.

Ladle into individual bowls and serve hot. Bon appétit!

Winter Quinoa Salad with Pickles

(Ready in about 20 minutes + chilling time | Servings 4)

Per serving : Calories: 346; Fat: 16.7g; Carbs: 42.6g; Protein: 9.3g

Ingredients

1 cup quinoa

4 garlic cloves, minced

2 pickled cucumber, chopped

10 ounces canned red peppers, chopped

1/2 cup green olives, pitted and sliced

2 cups green cabbages, shredded

2 cups Iceberg lettuce, torn into pieces

4 pickled chilies, chopped

4 tablespoons olive oil

1 tablespoon lemon juice

1 teaspoon lemon zest

1/2 teaspoon dried marjoram

Sea salt and ground black pepper, to taste

1/4 cup fresh chives, coarsely chopped

Directions

Place two cups of water and the quinoa in a pot and bring it to a boil. Immediately turn the heat to a simmer.

Let it simmer for about 13 minutes until the quinoa has absorbed all of the water; fluff the quinoa with a fork and let it cool completely. Then, transfer the quinoa to a salad bowl.

Add the garlic, pickled cucumber, peppers, olives, cabbage, lettuce and pickled chilies to the salad bowl and toss to combine.

In a small mixing bowl, make the dressing by whisking the remaining ingredients. Dress the salad, toss to combine well and serve immediately. Bon appétit!

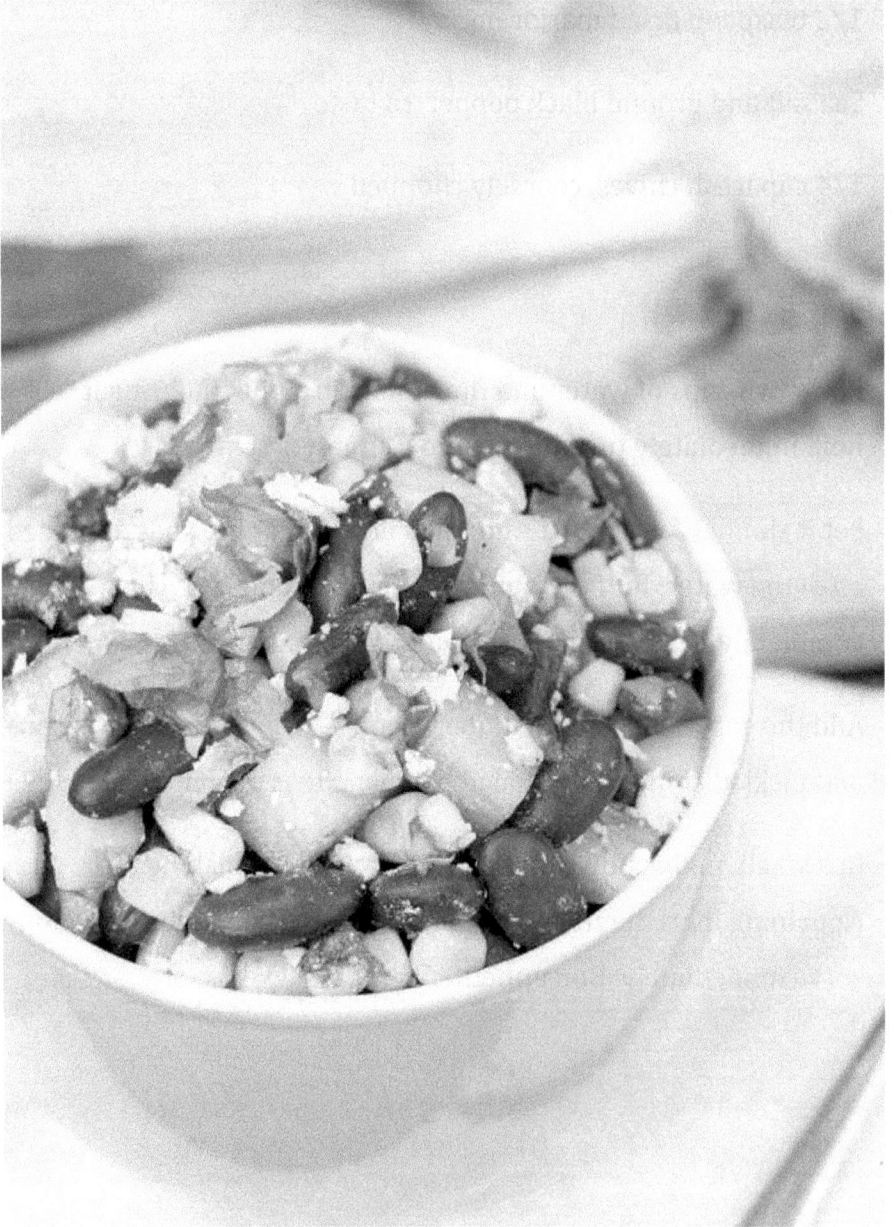

Roasted Wild Mushroom Soup

(Ready in about 55 minutes | Servings 3)

Per serving : Calories: 313; Fat: 23.5g; Carbs: 14.5g; Protein: 14.5g

Ingredients

3 tablespoons sesame oil

1 pound mixed wild mushrooms, sliced

1 white onion, chopped

3 cloves garlic, minced and divided

2 sprigs thyme, chopped

2 sprigs rosemary, chopped

1/4 cup flaxseed meal

1/4 cup dry white wine

3 cups vegetable broth

1/2 teaspoon red chili flakes

Garlic salt and freshly ground black pepper, to seasoned

Directions

Start by preheating your oven to 395 degrees F.

Place the mushrooms in a single layer onto a parchment-lined baking pan. Drizzle the mushrooms with 1 tablespoon of the sesame oil.

Roast the mushrooms in the preheated oven for about 25 minutes, or until tender.

Heat the remaining 2 tablespoons of the sesame oil in a stockpot over medium heat. Then, sauté the onion for about 3 minutes or until tender and translucent.

Then, add in the garlic, thyme and rosemary and continue to sauté for 1 minute or so until aromatic. Sprinkle flaxseed meal over everything.

Add in the remaining ingredients and continue to simmer for 10 to 15 minutes longer or until everything is cooked through.

Stir in the roasted mushrooms and continue simmering for a further 12 minutes. Ladle into soup bowls and serve hot. Enjoy!

Mediterranean-Style Green Bean Soup

(Ready in about 25 minutes | Servings 5)

Per serving : Calories: 313; Fat: 23.5g; Carbs: 14.5g; Protein: 14.5g

Ingredients

2 tablespoons olive oil

1 onion, chopped

1 celery with leaves, chopped

1 carrot, chopped

2 garlic cloves, minced

1 zucchini, chopped

5 cups vegetable broth

1 ¼ pounds green beans, trimmed and cut into bite-sized chunks

2 medium-sized tomatoes, pureed

Sea salt and freshly ground black pepper, to taste

1/2 teaspoon cayenne pepper

1 teaspoon oregano

1/2 teaspoon dried dill

1/2 cup Kalamata olives, pitted and sliced

Directions

In a heavy-bottomed pot, heat the olive over medium-high heat. Now, sauté the onion, celery and carrot for about 4 minutes or until the vegetables are just tender.

Add in the garlic and zucchini and continue to sauté for 1 minute or until aromatic.

Then, stir in the vegetable broth, green beans, tomatoes, salt, black pepper, cayenne pepper, oregano and dried dill; bring to a boil. Immediately reduce the heat to a simmer and let it cook for about 15 minutes.

Ladle into individual bowls and serve with sliced olives. Bon appétit!

Cream of Carrot Soup

(Ready in about 30 minutes | Servings 4)

Per serving : Calories: 333; Fat: 23g; Carbs: 26g; Protein: 8.5g

Ingredients

2 tablespoons sesame oil

1 onion, chopped

1 ½ pounds carrots, trimmed and chopped

1 parsnip, chopped

2 garlic cloves, minced

1/2 teaspoon curry powder

Sea salt and cayenne pepper, to taste

4 cups vegetable broth

1 cup full-fat coconut milk

Directions

In a heavy-bottomed pot, heat the sesame oil over medium-high heat. Now, sauté the onion, carrots and parsnip for about 5 minutes, stirring periodically.

Add in the garlic and continue sautéing for 1 minute or until fragrant.

Then, stir in the curry powder, salt, cayenne pepper and vegetable broth; bring to a rapid boil. Immediately reduce the heat to a simmer and let it cook for 18 to 20 minutes.

Puree the soup using an immersion blender until creamy and uniform.

Return the pureed mixture to the pot. Fold in the coconut milk and continue to simmer until heated through or about 5 minutes longer.

Ladle into four bowls and serve hot. Bon appétit!

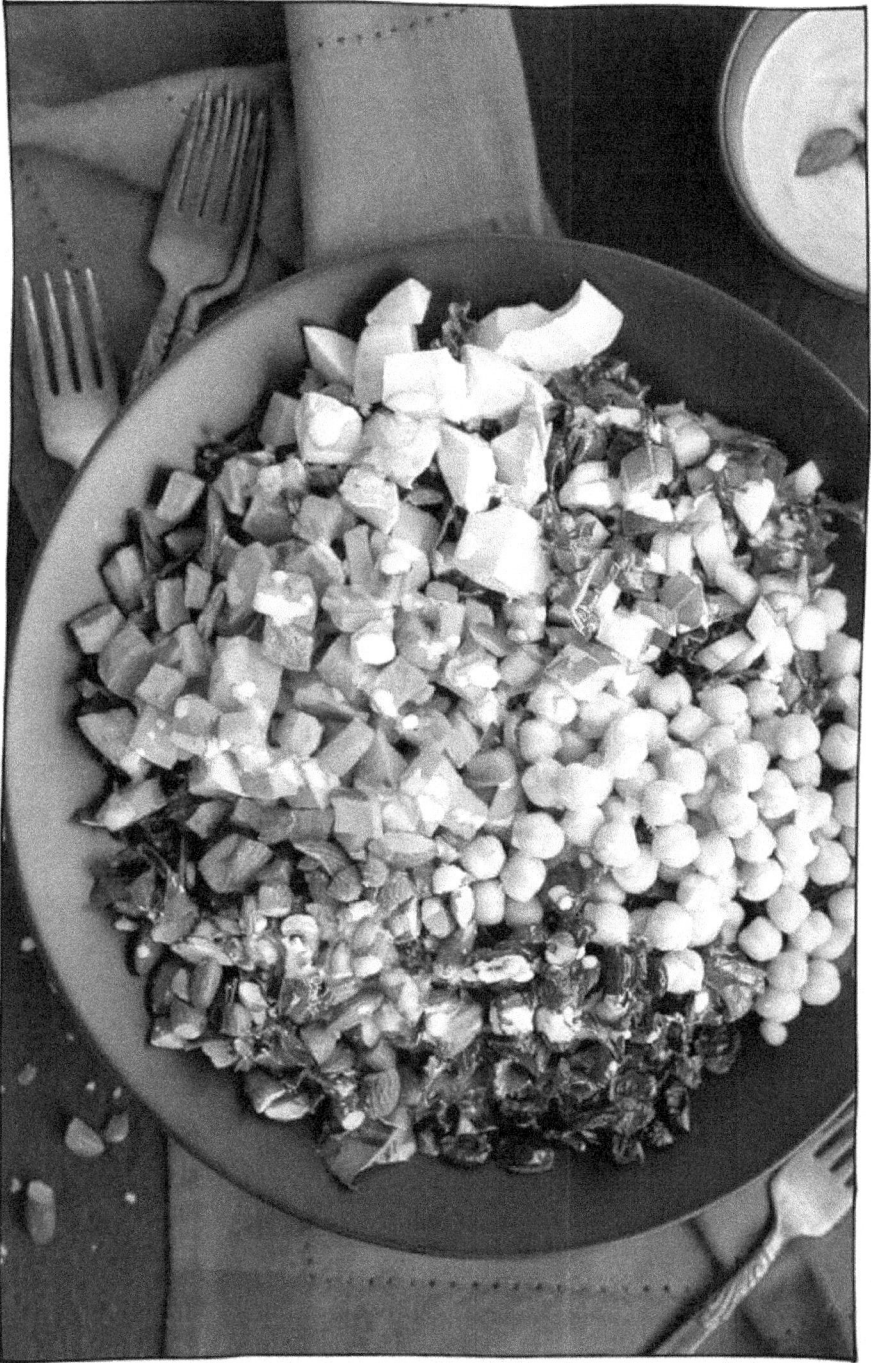

Italian Nonna's Pizza Salad

(Ready in about 15 minutes + chilling time | Servings 4)

Per serving : Calories: 595; Fat: 17.2g; Carbs: 93g; Protein: 16g

Ingredients

1 pound macaroni

1 cup marinated mushrooms, sliced

1 cup grape tomatoes, halved

4 tablespoons scallions, chopped

1 teaspoon garlic, minced

1 Italian pepper, sliced

1/4 cup extra-virgin olive oil

1/4 cup balsamic vinegar

1 teaspoon dried oregano

1 teaspoon dried basil

1/2 teaspoon dried rosemary

Sea salt and cayenne pepper, to taste

1/2 cup black olives, sliced

Directions

Cook the pasta according to the package directions. Drain and rinse the pasta. Let it cool completely and then, transfer it to a salad bowl.

Then, add in the remaining ingredients and toss until the macaroni are well coated.

Taste and adjust the seasonings; place the pizza salad in your refrigerator until ready to use. Bon appétit!

Creamy Golden Veggie Soup

(Ready in about 45 minutes | Servings 4)

Per serving : Calories: 550; Fat: 27.2g; Carbs: 70.4g; Protein: 13.2g

Ingredients

2 tablespoons avocado oil

1 yellow onion, chopped

2 Yukon Gold potatoes, peeled and diced

2 pounds butternut squash, peeled, seeded and diced

1 parsnip, trimmed and sliced

1 teaspoon ginger-garlic paste

1 teaspoon turmeric powder

1 teaspoon fennel seeds

1/2 teaspoon chili powder

1/2 teaspoon pumpkin pie spice

Kosher salt and ground black pepper, to taste

3 cups vegetable stock

1 cup full-fat coconut milk

2 tablespoons pepitas

Directions

In a heavy-bottomed pot, heat the oil over medium-high heat. Now, sauté the onion, potatoes, butternut squash and parsnip for about 10 minutes, stirring periodically to ensure even cooking.

Add in the ginger-garlic paste and continue sautéing for 1 minute or until aromatic.

Then, stir in the turmeric powder, fennel seeds, chili powder, pumpkin pie spice, salt, black pepper and vegetable stock; bring to a boil. Immediately reduce the heat to a simmer and let it cook for about 25 minutes.

Puree the soup using an immersion blender until creamy and uniform.

Return the pureed mixture to the pot. Fold in the coconut milk and continue to simmer until heated through or about 5 minutes longer.

Ladle into individual bowls and serve garnished with pepitas. Bon appétit!

Roasted Cauliflower Soup

(Ready in about 1 hour | Servings 4)

Per serving : Calories: 310; Fat: 24g; Carbs: 16.8g; Protein: 11.8g

Ingredients

1 ½ pounds cauliflower florets

4 tablespoons olive oil

1 onion, chopped

2 cloves garlic, minced

1/2 teaspoon ginger, peeled and minced

1 teaspoon fresh rosemary, chopped

2 tablespoons fresh basil, chopped

2 tablespoons fresh parsley, chopped

4 cups vegetable stock

Sea salt and ground black pepper, to taste

1/2 teaspoon ground sumac

1/4 cup tahini

1 lemon, freshly squeezed

Directions

Begin by preheating the oven to 425 degrees F. Toss the cauliflower with 2 tablespoons of the olive oil and arrange them on a parchment-lined roasting pan.

Then, roast the cauliflower florets for about 30 minutes stirring, them once or twice to promote even cooking.

Meanwhile, in a heavy-bottomed pot, heat the remaining 2 tablespoons of the olive oil over medium-high heat. Now, sauté the onion for about 4 minutes until tender and translucent.

Add in the garlic, ginger, rosemary, basil and parsley and continue sautéing for 1 minute or until fragrant.

Then, stir in the vegetable stock, salt, black pepper and sumac and bring it to a boil. Immediately reduce the heat to a simmer and let it cook for about 20 to 22 minutes.

Puree the soup using an immersion blender until creamy and uniform.

Return the pureed mixture to the pot. Fold in the tahini and continue to simmer for about 5 minutes or until everything is thoroughly cooked.

Ladle into individual bowls, garnish with lemon juice and serve hot. Enjoy!

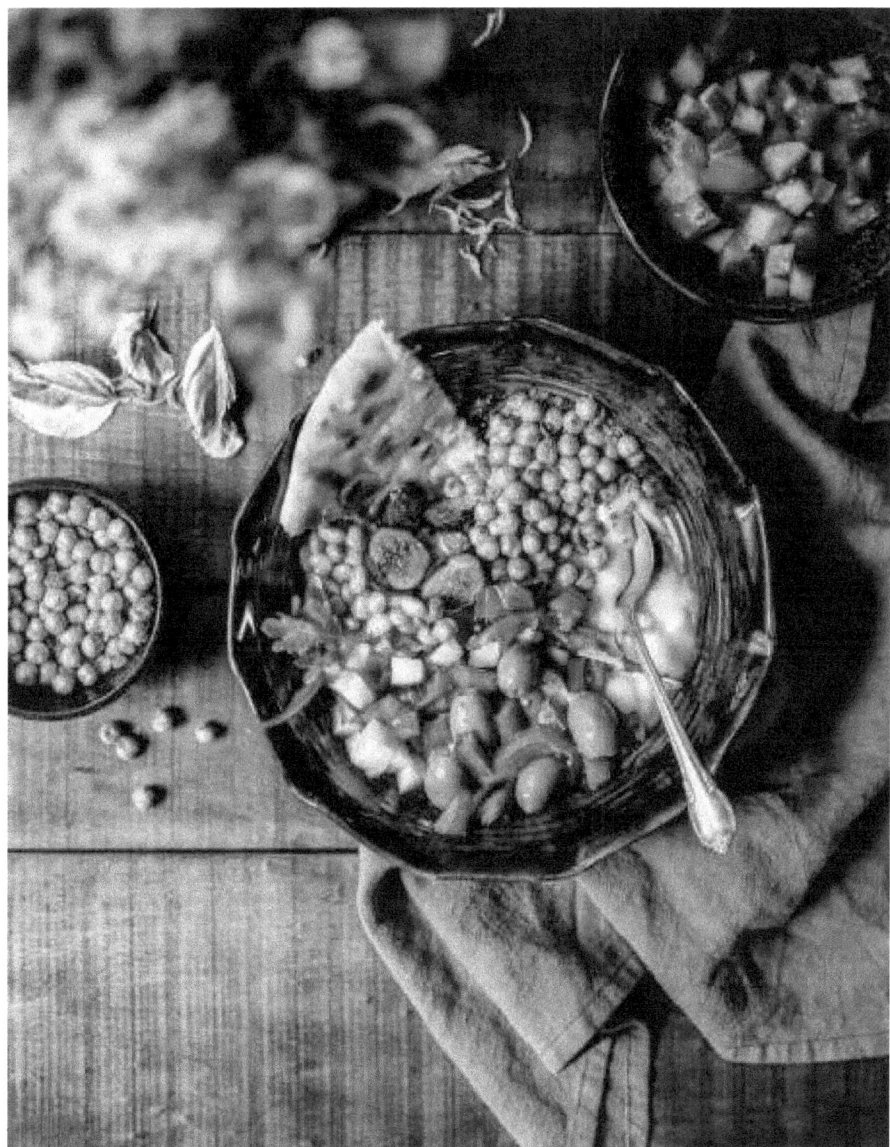

RICE & GRAINS

Classic Garlicky Rice

(Ready in about 20 minutes | Servings 4)

Per serving : Calories: 422; Fat: 15.1g; Carbs: 61.1g; Protein: 9.3g

Ingredients

4 tablespoons olive oil

4 cloves garlic, chopped

1 ½ cups white rice

2 ½ cups vegetable broth

Directions

In a saucepan, heat the olive oil over a moderately high flame. Add in the garlic and sauté for about 1 minute or until aromatic.

Add in the rice and broth. Bring to a boil; immediately turn the heat to a gentle simmer.

Cook for about 15 minutes or until all the liquid has absorbed. Fluff the rice with a fork, season with salt and pepper and serve hot!

Brown Rice with Vegetables and Tofu

(Ready in about 45 minutes | Servings 4)

Per serving : Calories: 410; Fat: 13.2g; Carbs: 60g; Protein: 14.3g

Ingredients

4 teaspoons sesame seeds

2 spring garlic stalks, minced

1 cup spring onions, chopped

1 carrot, trimmed and sliced

1 celery rib, sliced

1/4 cup dry white wine

10 ounces tofu, cubed

1 ½ cups long-grain brown rice, rinsed thoroughly

2 tablespoons soy sauce

2 tablespoons tahini

1 tablespoon lemon juice

Directions

In a wok or large saucepan, heat 2 teaspoons of the sesame oil over medium-high heat. Now, cook the garlic, onion, carrot and celery for about 3 minutes, stirring periodically to ensure even cooking.

Add the wine to deglaze the pan and push the vegetables to one side of the wok. Add in the remaining sesame oil and fry the tofu for 8 minutes, stirring occasionally.

Bring 2 ½ cups of water to a boil over medium-high heat. Bring to a simmer and cook the rice for about 30 minutes or until it is tender; fluff the rice and stir it with the soy sauce and tahini.

Stir the vegetables and tofu into the hot rice; add a few drizzles of the fresh lemon juice and serve warm. Bon appétit!

Basic Amaranth Porridge

(Ready in about 35 minutes | Servings 4)

Per serving : Calories: 261; Fat: 4.4g; Carbs: 49g; Protein: 7.3g

Ingredients

3 cups water

1 cup amaranth

1/2 cup coconut milk

4 tablespoons agave syrup

A pinch of kosher salt

A pinch of grated nutmeg

Directions

Bring the water to a boil over medium-high heat; add in the amaranth and turn the heat to a simmer.

Let it cook for about 30 minutes, stirring periodically to prevent the amaranth from sticking to the bottom of the pan.

Stir in the remaining ingredients and continue to cook for 1 to 2 minutes more until cooked through. Bon appétit!

. Country Cornbread with Spinach

(Ready in about 50 minutes | Servings 8)

Per serving : Calories: 282; Fat: 15.4g; Carbs: 30g; Protein: 4.6g

Ingredients

1 tablespoon flaxseed meal

1 cup all-purpose flour

1 cup yellow cornmeal

1/2 teaspoon baking soda

1/2 teaspoon baking powder

1 teaspoon kosher salt

1 teaspoon brown sugar

A pinch of grated nutmeg

1 ¼ cups oat milk, unsweetened

1 teaspoon white vinegar

1/2 cup olive oil

2 cups spinach, torn into pieces

Directions

Start by preheating your oven to 420 degrees F. Now, spritz a baking pan with a nonstick cooking spray.

To make the flax eggs, mix flaxseed meal with 3 tablespoons of the water. Stir and let it sit for about 15 minutes.

In a mixing bowl, thoroughly combine the flour, cornmeal, baking soda, baking powder, salt, sugar and grated nutmeg.

Gradually add in the flax egg, oat milk, vinegar and olive oil, whisking constantly to avoid lumps. Afterwards, fold in the spinach.

Scrape the batter into the prepared baking pan. Bake your cornbread for about 25 minutes or until a tester inserted in the middle comes out dry and clean.

Let it stand for about 10 minutes before slicing and serving. Bon appétit!

Rice Pudding with Currants

(Ready in about 45 minutes | Servings 4)

Per serving : Calories: 423; Fat: 5.3g; Carbs: 85g; Protein: 8.8g

Ingredients

1 ½ cups water

1 cup white rice

2 ½ cups oat milk, divided

1/2 cup white sugar

A pinch of salt

A pinch of grated nutmeg

1 teaspoon ground cinnamon

1/2 teaspoon vanilla extract

1/2 cup dried currants

Directions

In a saucepan, bring the water to a boil over medium-high heat. Immediately turn the heat to a simmer, add in the rice and let it cook for about 20 minutes.

Add in the milk, sugar and spices and continue to cook for 20 minutes more, stirring constantly to prevent the rice from sticking to the pan.

Top with dried currants and serve at room temperature. Bon appétit!

Millet Porridge with Sultanas

(Ready in about 25 minutes | Servings 3)

Per serving : Calories: 353; Fat: 5.5g; Carbs: 65.2g; Protein: 9.8g

Ingredients

1 cup water

1 cup coconut milk

1 cup millet, rinsed

1/4 teaspoon grated nutmeg

1/4 teaspoon ground cinnamon

1 teaspoon vanilla paste

1/4 teaspoon kosher salt

2 tablespoons agave syrup

4 tablespoons sultana raisins

Directions

Place the water, milk, millet, nutmeg, cinnamon, vanilla and salt in a saucepan; bring to a boil.

Turn the heat to a simmer and let it cook for about 20 minutes; fluff the millet with a fork and spoon into individual bowls.

Serve with agave syrup and sultanas. Bon appétit!

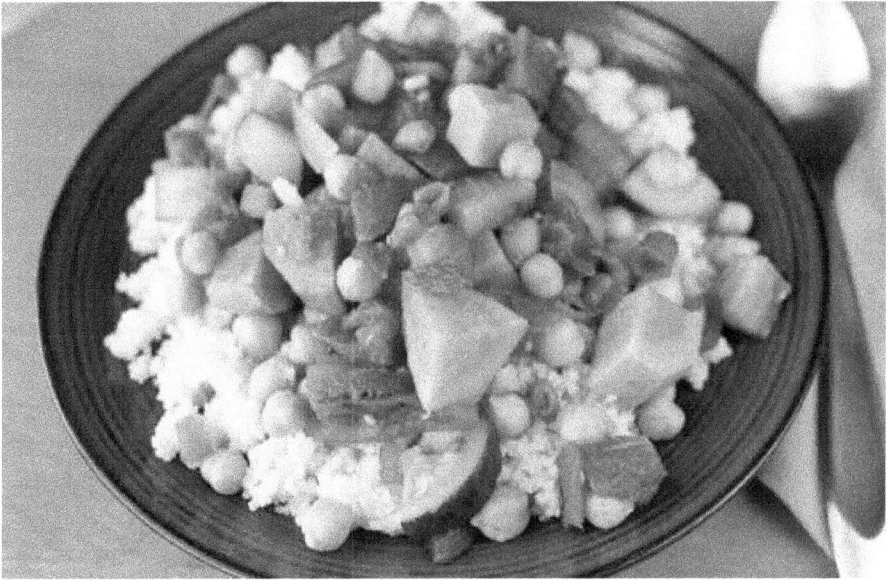

Quinoa Porridge with Dried Figs

(Ready in about 25 minutes | Servings 3)

Per serving : Calories: 414; Fat: 9g; Carbs: 71.2g; Protein: 13.8g

Ingredients

1 cup white quinoa, rinsed

2 cups almond milk

4 tablespoons brown sugar

A pinch of salt

1/4 teaspoon grated nutmeg

1/2 teaspoon ground cinnamon

1/2 teaspoon vanilla extract

1/2 cup dried figs, chopped

Directions

Place the quinoa, almond milk, sugar, salt, nutmeg, cinnamon and vanilla extract in a saucepan.

Bring it to a boil over medium-high heat. Turn the heat to a simmer and let it cook for about 20 minutes; fluff with a fork.

Divide between three serving bowls and garnish with dried figs. Bon appétit!

Bread Pudding with Raisins

(Ready in about 1 hour | Servings 4)

Per serving : Calories: 474; Fat: 12.2g; Carbs: 72g; Protein: 14.4g

Ingredients

4 cups day-old bread, cubed

1 cup brown sugar

4 cups coconut milk

1/2 teaspoon vanilla extract

1 teaspoon ground cinnamon

2 tablespoons rum

1/2 cup raisins

Directions

Start by preheating your oven to 360 degrees F. Lightly oil a casserole dish with a nonstick cooking spray.

Place the cubed bread in the prepared casserole dish.

In a mixing bowl, thoroughly combine the sugar, milk, vanilla, cinnamon, rum and raisins. Pour the custard evenly over the bread cubes.

Let it soak for about 15 minutes.

Bake in the preheated oven for about 45 minutes or until the top is golden and set. Bon appétit!

Bulgur Wheat Salad

(Ready in about 25 minutes | Servings 4)

Per serving : Calories: 359; Fat: 15.5g; Carbs: 48.1g; Protein: 10.1g

Ingredients

1 cup bulgur wheat

1 ½ cups vegetable broth

1 teaspoon sea salt

1 teaspoon fresh ginger, minced

4 tablespoons olive oil

1 onion, chopped

8 ounces canned garbanzo beans, drained

2 large roasted peppers, sliced

2 tablespoons fresh parsley, roughly chopped

Directions

In a deep saucepan, bring the bulgur wheat and vegetable broth to a simmer; let it cook, covered, for 12 to 13 minutes.

Let it stand for about 10 minutes and fluff with a fork.

Add the remaining ingredients to the cooked bulgur wheat; serve at room temperature or well-chilled. Bon appétit!

Rye Porridge with Blueberry Topping

(Ready in about 15 minutes | Servings 3)

Per serving : Calories: 359; Fat: 11g; Carbs: 56.1g; Protein: 12.1g

Ingredients

1 cup rye flakes

1 cup water

1 cup coconut milk

1 cup fresh blueberries

1 tablespoon coconut oil

6 dates, pitted

Directions

Add the rye flakes, water and coconut milk to a deep saucepan; bring to a boil over medium-high. Turn the heat to a simmer and let it cook for 5 to 6 minutes.

In a blender or food processor, puree the blueberries with the coconut oil and dates.

Ladle into three bowls and garnish with the blueberry topping.

Bon appétit!

Coconut Sorghum Porridge

(Ready in about 15 minutes | Servings 2)

Per serving : Calories: 289; Fat: 5.1g; Carbs: 57.8g; Protein: 7.3g

Ingredients

1/2 cup sorghum

1 cup water

1/2 cup coconut milk

1/4 teaspoon grated nutmeg

1/4 teaspoon ground cloves

1/2 teaspoon ground cinnamon

Kosher salt, to taste

2 tablespoons agave syrup

2 tablespoons coconut flakes

Directions

Place the sorghum, water, milk, nutmeg, cloves, cinnamon and kosher salt in a saucepan; simmer gently for about 15 minutes.

Spoon the porridge into serving bowls. Top with agave syrup and coconut flakes. Bon appétit!

Dad's Aromatic Rice

(Ready in about 20 minutes | Servings 4)

Per serving : Calories: 384; Fat: 11.4g; Carbs: 60.4g; Protein: 8.3g

Ingredients

3 tablespoons olive oil

1 teaspoon garlic, minced

1 teaspoon dried oregano

1 teaspoon dried rosemary

1 bay leaf

1 ½ cups white rice

2 ½ cups vegetable broth

Sea salt and cayenne pepper, to taste

Directions

In a saucepan, heat the olive oil over a moderately high flame. Add in the garlic, oregano, rosemary and bay leaf; sauté for about 1 minute or until aromatic.

Add in the rice and broth. Bring to a boil; immediately turn the heat to a gentle simmer.

Cook for about 15 minutes or until all the liquid has absorbed. Fluff the rice with a fork, season with salt and pepper and serve immediately.

Bon appétit!

Everyday Savory Grits

(Ready in about 35 minutes | Servings 4)

Per serving : Calories: 238; Fat: 6.5g; Carbs: 38.7g; Protein: 3.7g

Ingredients

2 tablespoons vegan butter

1 sweet onion, chopped

1 teaspoon garlic, minced

4 cups water

1 cup stone-ground grits

Sea salt and cayenne pepper, to taste

Directions

In a saucepan, melt the vegan butter over medium-high heat. Once hot, cook the onion for about 3 minutes or until tender.

Add in the garlic and continue to sauté for 30 seconds more or until aromatic; reserve.

Bring the water to a boil over a moderately high heat. Stir in the grits, salt and pepper. Turn the heat to a simmer, cover and continue to cook, for about 30 minutes or until cooked through.

Stir in the sautéed mixture and serve warm. Bon appétit!

Greek-Style Barley Salad

(Ready in about 35 minutes | Servings 4)

Per serving : Calories: 378; Fat: 15.6g; Carbs: 50g; Protein: 10.7g

Ingredients

1 cup pearl barley

2 ¾ cups vegetable broth

2 tablespoons apple cider vinegar

4 tablespoons extra-virgin olive oil

2 bell peppers, seeded and diced

1 shallot, chopped

2 ounces sun-dried tomatoes in oil, chopped

1/2 green olives, pitted and sliced

2 tablespoons fresh cilantro, roughly chopped

Directions

Bring the barley and broth to a boil over medium-high heat; now, turn the heat to a simmer.

Continue to simmer for about 30 minutes until all the liquid has absorbed; fluff with a fork.

Toss the barley with the vinegar, olive oil, peppers, shallots, sun-dried tomatoes and olives; toss to combine well.

Garnish with fresh cilantro and serve at room temperature or well-chilled. Enjoy!

Easy Sweet Maize Meal Porridge

(Ready in about 15 minutes | Servings 2)

Per serving : Calories: 278; Fat: 12.7g; Carbs: 37.2g; Protein: 3g

Ingredients

2 cups water

1/2 cup maize meal

1/4 teaspoon ground allspice

1/4 teaspoon salt

2 tablespoons brown sugar

2 tablespoons almond butter

Directions

In a saucepan, bring the water to a boil; then, gradually add in the maize meal and turn the heat to a simmer.

Add in the ground allspice and salt. Let it cook for 10 minutes.

Add in the brown sugar and almond butter and gently stir to combine. Bon appétit!

Mom's Millet Muffins

(Ready in about 20 minutes | Servings 8)

Per serving : Calories: 367; Fat: 15.9g; Carbs: 53.7g; Protein: 6.5g

Ingredients

2 cup whole-wheat flour

1/2 cup millet

2 teaspoons baking powder

1/2 teaspoon salt

1 cup coconut milk

1/2 cup coconut oil, melted

1/2 cup agave nectar

1/2 teaspoon ground cinnamon

1/4 teaspoon ground cloves

A pinch of grated nutmeg

1/2 cup dried apricots, chopped

Directions

Begin by preheating your oven to 400 degrees F. Lightly oil a muffin tin with a nonstick oil.

In a mixing bowl, mix all dry ingredients. In a separate bowl, mix the wet ingredients. Stir the milk mixture into the flour mixture; mix just until evenly moist and do not overmix your batter.

Fold in the apricots and scrape the batter into the prepared muffin cups.

Bake the muffins in the preheated oven for about 15 minutes, or until a tester inserted in the center of your muffin comes out dry and clean.

Let it stand for 10 minutes on a wire rack before unmolding and serving. Enjoy!

Ginger Brown Rice

(Ready in about 30 minutes | Servings 4)

Per serving : Calories: 318; Fat: 8.8g; Carbs: 53.4g; Protein: 5.6g

Ingredients

1 ½ cups brown rice, rinsed

2 tablespoons olive oil

1 teaspoon garlic, minced

1 (1-inch) piece ginger, peeled and minced

1/2 teaspoon cumin seeds

Sea salt and ground black pepper, to taste

Directions

Place the brown rice in a saucepan and cover with cold water by 2 inches. Bring to a boil.

Turn the heat to a simmer and continue to cook for about 30 minutes or until tender.

In a sauté pan, heat the olive oil over medium-high heat. Once hot, cook the garlic, ginger and cumin seeds until aromatic.

Stir the garlic/ginger mixture into the hot rice; season with salt and pepper and serve immediately. Bon appétit!

Sweet Oatmeal "Grits"

(Ready in about 20 minutes | Servings 4)

Per serving : Calories: 380; Fat: 11.1g; Carbs: 59g; Protein: 14.4g

Ingredients

1 ½ cups steel-cut oats, soaked overnight

1 cup almond milk

2 cups water

A pinch of grated nutmeg

A pinch of ground cloves

A pinch of sea salt

4 tablespoons almonds, slivered

6 dates, pitted and chopped

6 prunes, chopped

Directions

In a deep saucepan, bring the steel cut oats, almond milk and water to a boil.

Add in the nutmeg, cloves and salt. Immediately turn the heat to a simmer, cover and continue to cook for about 15 minutes or until they've softened.

Then, spoon the grits into four serving bowls; top them with the almonds, dates and prunes.

Bon appétit!

Freekeh Bowl with Dried Figs

(Ready in about 35 minutes | Servings 2)

Per serving : Calories: 458; Fat: 6.8g; Carbs: 90g; Protein: 12.4g

Ingredients

1/2 cup freekeh, soaked for 30 minutes, drained

1 1/3 cups almond milk

1/4 teaspoon sea salt

1/4 teaspoon ground cloves

1/4 teaspoon ground cinnamon

4 tablespoons agave syrup

2 ounces dried figs, chopped

Directions

Place the freekeh, milk, sea salt, ground cloves and cinnamon in a saucepan. Bring to a boil over medium-high heat.

Immediately turn the heat to a simmer for 30 to 35 minutes, stirring occasionally to promote even cooking.

Stir in the agave syrup and figs. Ladle the porridge into individual bowls and serve. Bon appétit!

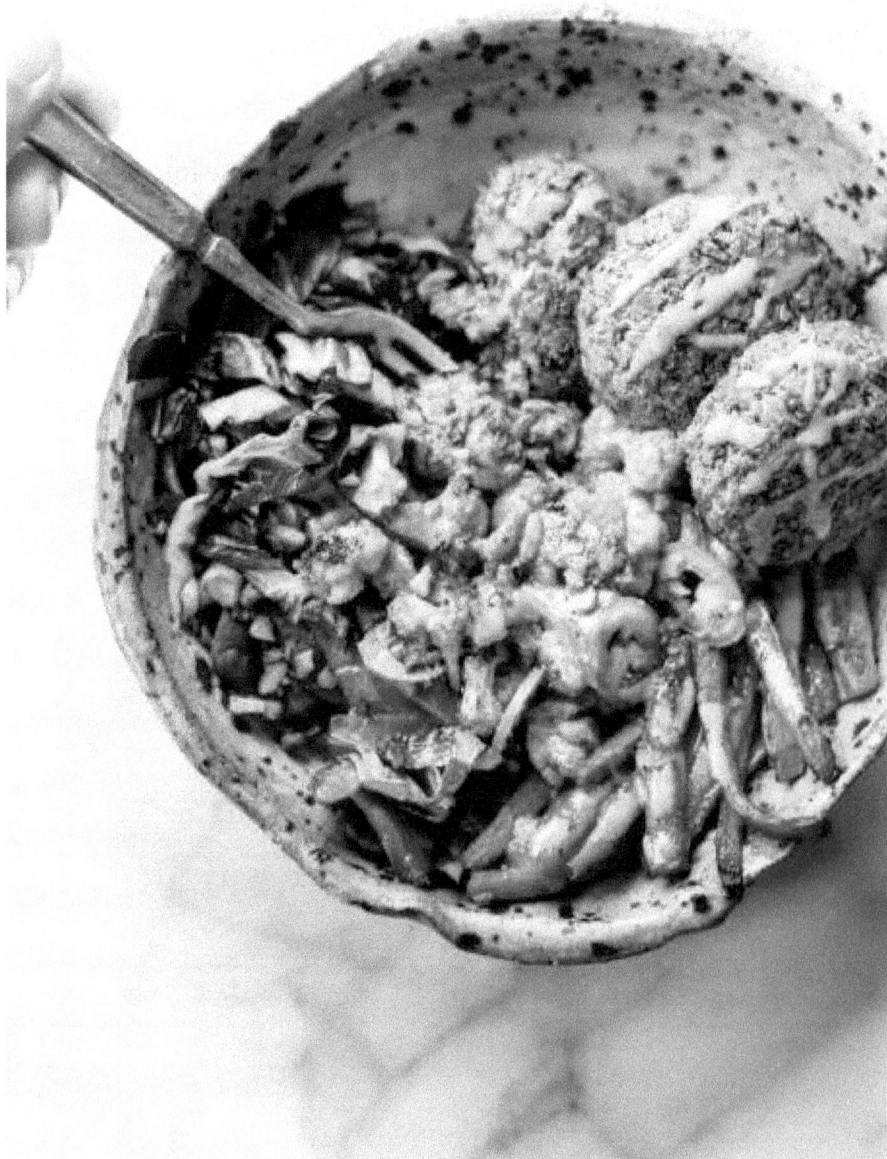

Cornmeal Porridge with Maple Syrup

(Ready in about 20 minutes | Servings 4)

Per serving : Calories: 328; Fat: 4.8g; Carbs: 63.4g; Protein: 6.6g

Ingredients

2 cups water

2 cups almond milk

1 cinnamon stick

1 vanilla bean

1 cup yellow cornmeal

1/2 cup maple syrup

Directions

In a saucepan, bring the water and almond milk to a boil. Add in the cinnamon stick and vanilla bean.

Gradually add in the cornmeal, stirring continuously; turn the heat to a simmer. Let it simmer for about 15 minutes.

Drizzle the maple syrup over the porridge and serve warm. Enjoy!

Mediterranean-Style Rice

(Ready in about 20 minutes | Servings 4)

Per serving : Calories: 403; Fat: 12g; Carbs: 64.1g; Protein: 8.3g

Ingredients

3 tablespoons vegan butter, at room temperature

4 tablespoons scallions, chopped

2 cloves garlic, minced

1 bay leaf

1 thyme sprig, chopped

1 rosemary sprig, chopped

1 ½ cups white rice

2 cups vegetable broth

1 large tomato, pureed

Sea salt and ground black pepper, to taste

2 ounces Kalamata olives, pitted and sliced

Directions

In a saucepan, melt the vegan butter over a moderately high flame. Cook the scallions for about 2 minutes or until tender.

Add in the garlic, bay leaf, thyme and rosemary and continue to sauté for about 1 minute or until aromatic.

Add in the rice, broth and pureed tomato. Bring to a boil; immediately turn the heat to a gentle simmer.

Cook for about 15 minutes or until all the liquid has absorbed. Fluff the rice with a fork, season with salt and pepper and garnish with olives; serve immediately.

Bon appétit!

Bulgur Pancakes with a Twist

(Ready in about 50 minutes | Servings 4)

Per serving : Calories: 414; Fat: 21.8g; Carbs: 51.8g; Protein: 6.5g

Ingredients

1/2 cup bulgur wheat flour

1/2 cup almond flour

1 teaspoon baking soda

1/2 teaspoon fine sea salt

1 cup full-fat coconut milk

1/2 teaspoon ground cinnamon

1/4 teaspoon ground cloves

4 tablespoons coconut oil

1/2 cup maple syrup

1 large-sized banana, sliced

Directions

In a mixing bowl, thoroughly combine the flour, baking soda, salt, coconut milk, cinnamon and ground cloves; let it stand for 30 minutes to soak well.

Heat a small amount of the coconut oil in a frying pan.

Fry the pancakes until the surface is golden brown. Garnish with maple syrup and banana. Bon appétit!

Chocolate Rye Porridge

(Ready in about 10 minutes | Servings 4)

Per serving : Calories: 460; Fat: 13.1g; Carbs: 72.2g; Protein: 15g

Ingredients

2 cups rye flakes

2 ½ cups almond milk

2 ounces dried prunes, chopped

2 ounces dark chocolate chunks

Directions

Add the rye flakes and almond milk to a deep saucepan; bring to a boil over medium-high. Turn the heat to a simmer and let it cook for 5 to 6 minutes.

Remove from the heat. Fold in the chopped prunes and chocolate chunks, gently stir to combine.

Ladle into serving bowls and serve warm.

Bon appétit!

Authentic African Mielie-Meal

(Ready in about 15 minutes | Servings 4)

Per serving : Calories: 336; Fat: 15.1g; Carbs: 47.9g; Protein: 4.1g

Ingredients

3 cups water

1 cup coconut milk

1 cup maize meal

1/3 teaspoon kosher salt

1/4 teaspoon grated nutmeg

1/4 teaspoon ground cloves

4 tablespoons maple syrup

Directions

In a saucepan, bring the water and milk to a boil; then, gradually add in the maize meal and turn the heat to a simmer.

Add in the salt, nutmeg and cloves. Let it cook for 10 minutes.

Add in the maple syrup and gently stir to combine. Bon appétit!

Teff Porridge with Dried Figs

(Ready in about 25 minutes | Servings 4)

Per serving : Calories: 356; Fat: 12.1g; Carbs: 56.5g; Protein: 6.8g

Ingredients

1 cup whole-grain teff

1 cup water

2 cups coconut milk

2 tablespoons coconut oil

1/2 teaspoon ground cardamom

1/4 teaspoon ground cinnamon

4 tablespoons agave syrup

7-8 dried figs, chopped

Directions

Bring the whole-grain teff, water and coconut milk to a boil.

Turn the heat to a simmer and add in the coconut oil, cardamom and cinnamon.

Let it cook for 20 minutes or until the grain has softened and the porridge has thickened. Stir in the agave syrup and stir to combine well.

Top each serving bowl with chopped figs and serve warm. Bon appétit!

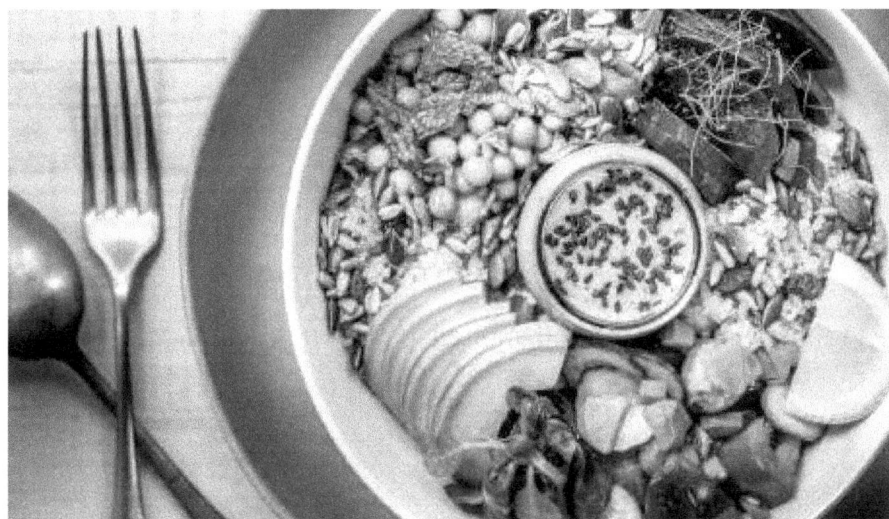

Decadent Bread Pudding with Apricots

(Ready in about 1 hour | Servings 4)

Per serving : Calories: 418; Fat: 18.8g; Carbs: 56.9g; Protein: 7.3g

Ingredients

4 cups day-old ciabatta bread, cubed

4 tablespoons coconut oil, melted

2 cups coconut milk

1/2 cup coconut sugar

4 tablespoons applesauce

1/4 teaspoon ground cloves

1/2 teaspoon ground cinnamon

1 teaspoon vanilla extract

1/3 cup dried apricots, diced

Directions

Start by preheating your oven to 360 degrees F. Lightly oil a casserole dish with a nonstick cooking spray.

Place the cubed bread in the prepared casserole dish.

In a mixing bowl, thoroughly combine the coconut oil, milk, coconut sugar, applesauce, ground cloves, ground cinnamon and vanilla. Pour the custard evenly over the bread cubes; fold in the apricots.

Press with a wide spatula and let it soak for about 15 minutes.

Bake in the preheated oven for about 45 minutes or until the top is golden and set. Bon appétit!

Chipotle Cilantro Rice

(Ready in about 25 minutes | Servings 4)

Per serving : Calories: 313; Fat: 15g; Carbs: 37.1g; Protein: 5.7g

Ingredients

4 tablespoons olive oil

1 chipotle pepper, seeded and chopped

1 cup jasmine rice

1 ½ cups vegetable broth

1/4 cup fresh cilantro, chopped

Sea salt and cayenne pepper, to taste

Directions

In a saucepan, heat the olive oil over a moderately high flame. Add in the pepper and rice and cook for about 3 minutes or until aromatic.

Pour the vegetable broth into the saucepan and bring to a boil; immediately turn the heat to a gentle simmer.

Cook for about 18 minutes or until all the liquid has absorbed. Fluff the rice with a fork, add in the cilantro, salt and cayenne pepper; stir to combine well. Bon appétit!

Oat Porridge with Almonds

(Ready in about 20 minutes | Servings 2)

Per serving : Calories: 533; Fat: 13.7g; Carbs: 85g; Protein: 21.6g

Ingredients

1 cup water

2 cups almond milk, divided

1 cup rolled oats

2 tablespoons coconut sugar

1/2 vanilla essence

1/4 teaspoon cardamom

1/2 cup almonds, chopped

1 banana, sliced

Directions

In a deep saucepan, bring the water and milk to a rapid boil. Add in the oats, cover the saucepan and turn the heat to medium.

Add in the coconut sugar, vanilla and cardamom. Continue to cook for about 12 minutes, stirring periodically.

Spoon the mixture into serving bowls; top with almonds and banana. Bon appétit!

Aromatic Millet Bowl

(Ready in about 20 minutes | Servings 3)

Per serving : Calories: 363; Fat: 6.7g; Carbs: 63.5g; Protein: 11.6g

Ingredients

1 cup water

1 ½ cups coconut milk

1 cup millet, rinsed and drained

1/4 teaspoon crystallized ginger

1/4 teaspoon ground cinnamon

A pinch of grated nutmeg

A pinch of Himalayan salt

2 tablespoons maple syrup

Directions

Place the water, milk, millet, crystallized ginger cinnamon, nutmeg and salt in a saucepan; bring to a boil.

Turn the heat to a simmer and let it cook for about 20 minutes; fluff the millet with a fork and spoon into individual bowls.

Serve with maple syrup. Bon appétit!

Harissa Bulgur Bowl

(Ready in about 25 minutes | Servings 4)

Per serving : Calories: 353; Fat: 15.5g; Carbs: 48.5g; Protein: 8.4g

Ingredients

1 cup bulgur wheat

1 ½ cups vegetable broth

2 cups sweet corn kernels, thawed

1 cup canned kidney beans, drained

1 red onion, thinly sliced

1 garlic clove, minced

Sea salt and ground black pepper, to taste

1/4 cup harissa paste

1 tablespoon lemon juice

1 tablespoon white vinegar

1/4 cup extra-virgin olive oil

1/4 cup fresh parsley leaves, roughly chopped

Directions

In a deep saucepan, bring the bulgur wheat and vegetable broth to a simmer; let it cook, covered, for 12 to 13 minutes.

Let it stand for 5 to 10 minutes and fluff your bulgur with a fork.

Add the remaining ingredients to the cooked bulgur wheat; serve warm or at room temperature. Bon appétit!

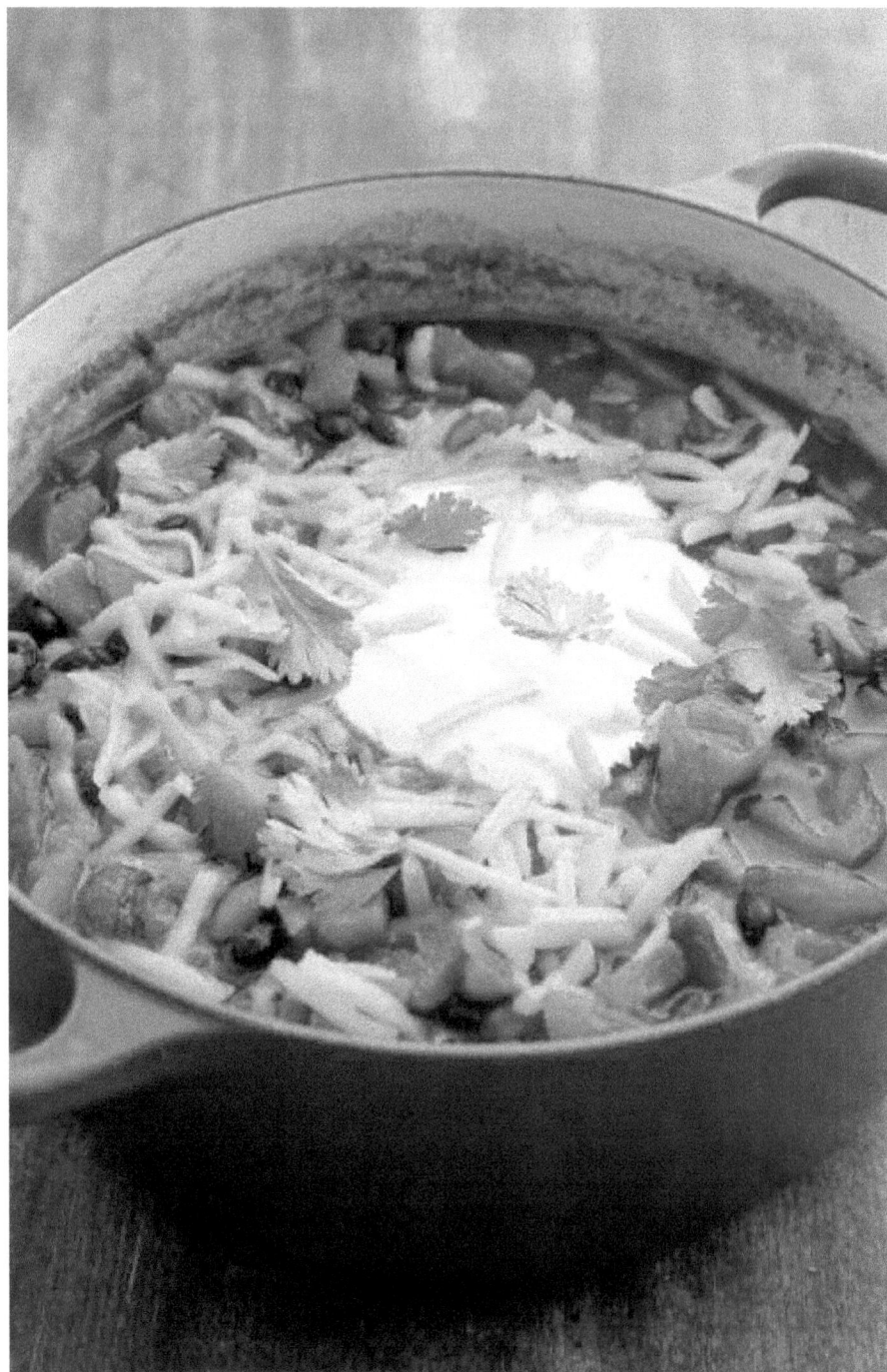

Coconut Quinoa Pudding

(Ready in about 20 minutes | Servings 3)

Per serving : Calories: 391; Fat: 10.6g; Carbs: 65.2g; Protein: 11.1g

Ingredients

1 cup water

1 cup coconut milk

1 cup quinoa

A pinch of kosher salt

A pinch of ground allspice

1/2 teaspoon cinnamon

1/2 teaspoon vanilla extract

4 tablespoons agave syrup

1/2 cup coconut flakes

Directions

Place the water, coconut milk, quinoa, salt, ground allspice, cinnamon and vanilla extract in a saucepan.

Bring it to a boil over medium-high heat. Turn the heat to a simmer and let it cook for about 20 minutes; fluff with a fork and add in the agave syrup.

Divide between three serving bowls and garnish with coconut flakes. Bon appétit!

Cremini Mushroom Risotto

(Ready in about 20 minutes | Servings 3)

Per serving : Calories: 513; Fat: 12.5g; Carbs: 88g; Protein: 11.7g

Ingredients

3 tablespoons vegan butter

1 teaspoon garlic, minced

1 teaspoon thyme

1 pound Cremini mushrooms, sliced

1 ½ cups white rice

2 ½ cups vegetable broth

1/4 cup dry sherry wine

Kosher salt and ground black pepper, to taste

3 tablespoons fresh scallions, thinly sliced

Directions

In a saucepan, melt the vegan butter over a moderately high flame. Cook the garlic and thyme for about 1 minute or until aromatic.

Add in the mushrooms and continue to sauté until they release the liquid or about 3 minutes.

Add in the rice, vegetable broth and sherry wine. Bring to a boil; immediately turn the heat to a gentle simmer.

Cook for about 15 minutes or until all the liquid has absorbed. Fluff the rice with a fork, season with salt and pepper and garnish with fresh scallions.

Bon appétit!

Colorful Risotto with Vegetables

(Ready in about 35 minutes | Servings 5)

Per serving : Calories: 363; Fat: 7.5g; Carbs: 66.3g; Protein: 7.7g

Ingredients

2 tablespoons sesame oil

1 onion, chopped

2 bell peppers, chopped

1 parsnip, trimmed and chopped

1 carrot, trimmed and chopped

1 cup broccoli florets

2 garlic cloves, finely chopped

1/2 teaspoon ground cumin

2 cups brown rice

Sea salt and black pepper, to taste

1/2 teaspoon ground turmeric

2 tablespoons fresh cilantro, finely chopped

Directions

Heat the sesame oil in a saucepan over medium-high heat.

Once hot, cook the onion, peppers, parsnip, carrot and broccoli for about 3 minutes until aromatic.

Add in the garlic and ground cumin; continue to cook for 30 seconds more until aromatic.

Place the brown rice in a saucepan and cover with cold water by 2 inches. Bring to a boil. Turn the heat to a simmer and continue to cook for about 30 minutes or until tender.

Stir the rice into the vegetable mixture; season with salt, black pepper and ground turmeric; garnish with fresh cilantro and serve immediately. Bon appétit!

Amarant Grits with Walnuts

(Ready in about 35 minutes | Servings 4)

Per serving : Calories: 356; Fat: 12g; Carbs: 51.3g; Protein: 12.2g

Ingredients

2 cups water

2 cups coconut milk

1 cup amaranth

1 cinnamon stick

1 vanilla bean

4 tablespoons maple syrup

4 tablespoons walnuts, chopped

Directions

Bring the water and coconut milk to a boil over medium-high heat; add in the amaranth, cinnamon and vanilla and turn the heat to a simmer.

Let it cook for about 30 minutes, stirring periodically to prevent the amaranth from sticking to the bottom of the pan.

Top with maple syrup and walnuts. Bon appétit!

Barley Pilaf with Wild Mushrooms

(Ready in about 45 minutes | Servings 4)

Per serving : Calories: 288; Fat: 7.7g; Carbs: 45.3g; Protein: 12.1g

Ingredients

2 tablespoons vegan butter

1 small onion, chopped

1 teaspoon garlic, minced

1 jalapeno pepper, seeded and minced

1 pound wild mushrooms, sliced

1 cup medium pearl barley, rinsed

2 ¾ cups vegetable broth

Directions

Melt the vegan butter in a saucepan over medium-high heat.

Once hot, cook the onion for about 3 minutes until just tender.

Add in the garlic, jalapeno pepper, mushrooms; continue to sauté for 2 minutes or until aromatic.

Add in the barley and broth, cover and continue to simmer for about 30 minutes. Once all the liquid has absorbed, allow the barley to rest for about 10 minutes fluff with a fork.

Taste and adjust the seasonings. Bon appétit!

Sweet Cornbread Muffins

(Ready in about 30 minutes | Servings 8)

Per serving : Calories: 311; Fat: 13.7g; Carbs: 42.3g; Protein: 4.5g

Ingredients

1 cup all-purpose flour

1 cup yellow cornmeal

1 teaspoon baking powder

1 teaspoon baking soda

1 teaspoon kosher salt

1/2 cup sugar

1/2 teaspoon ground cinnamon

1 1/2 cups almond milk

1/2 cup vegan butter, melted

2 tablespoons applesauce

Directions

Start by preheating your oven to 420 degrees F. Now, spritz a muffin tin with a nonstick cooking spray.

In a mixing bowl, thoroughly combine the flour, cornmeal, baking soda, baking powder, salt, sugar and cinnamon.

Gradually add in the milk, butter and applesauce, whisking constantly to avoid lumps.

Scrape the batter into the prepared muffin tin. Bake your muffins for about 25 minutes or until a tester inserted in the middle comes out dry and clean.

Transfer them to a wire rack to rest for 5 minutes before unmolding and serving. Bon appétit!

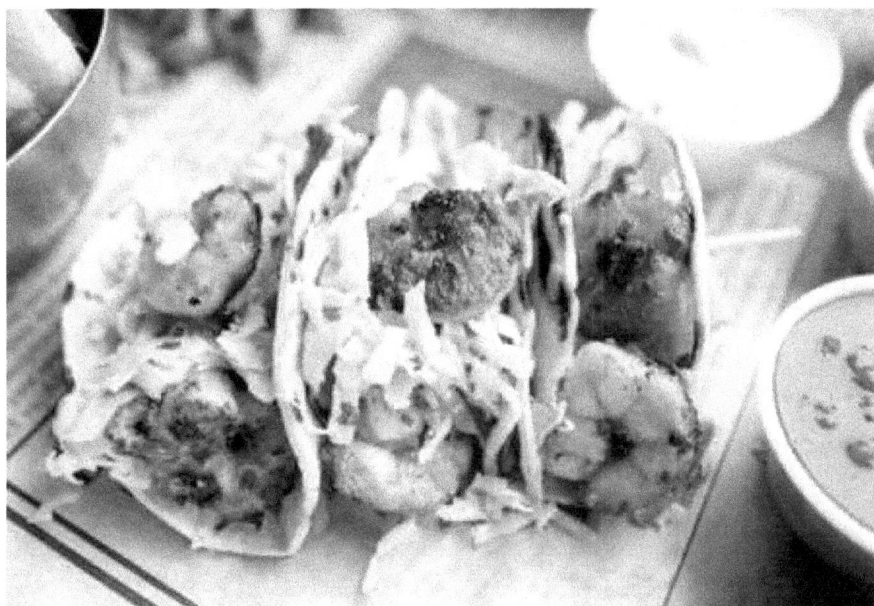

Aromatic Rice Pudding with Dried Figs

(Ready in about 45 minutes | Servings 4)

Per serving : Calories: 407; Fat: 7.5g; Carbs: 74.3g; Protein: 10.7g

Ingredients

2 cups water

1 cup medium-grain white rice

3 ½ cups coconut milk

1/2 cup coconut sugar

1 cinnamon stick

1 vanilla bean

1/2 cup dried figs, chopped

4 tablespoons coconut, shredded

Directions

In a saucepan, bring the water to a boil over medium-high heat. Immediately turn the heat to a simmer, add in the rice and let it cook for about 20 minutes.

Add in the milk, sugar and spices and continue to cook for 20 minutes more, stirring constantly to prevent the rice from sticking to the pan.

Top with dried figs and coconut; serve your pudding warm or at room temperature. Bon appétit!

Potage au Quinoa

(Ready in about 25 minutes | Servings 4)

Per serving : Calories: 466; Fat: 11.1g; Carbs: 76g; Protein: 16.1g

Ingredients

2 tablespoons olive oil

1 onion, chopped

4 medium potatoes, peeled and diced

1 carrot, trimmed and diced

1 parsnip, trimmed and diced

1 jalapeno pepper, seeded and chopped

4 cups vegetable broth

1 cup quinoa

Sea salt and ground white pepper, to taste

Directions

In a heavy-bottomed pot, heat the olive oil over medium-high heat. Sauté the onion, potatoes, carrots, parsnip and pepper for about 5 minutes or until they've softened.

Add in the vegetable broth and quinoa; bring to a boil.

Immediately turn the heat to a simmer for about 15 minutes or until the quinoa is tender.

Season with salt and pepper to taste. Puree your potage with an immersion blender. Reheat the potage just before serving and enjoy!

Sorghum Bowl with Almonds

(Ready in about 15 minutes | Servings 4)

Per serving : Calories: 384; Fat: 14.7g; Carbs: 54.6g; Protein: 13.9g

Ingredients

1 cup sorghum

3 cups almond milk

A pinch of sea salt

A pinch of grated nutmeg

1/2 teaspoon ground cinnamon

1/4 teaspoon ground cardamom

1 teaspoon crystallized ginger

4 tablespoons brown sugar

4 tablespoons almonds, slivered

Directions

Place the sorghum, almond milk, salt, nutmeg, cinnamon, cardamom and crystallized ginger in a saucepan; simmer gently for about 15 minutes.

Add in the brown sugar, stir and spoon the porridge into serving bowls.

Top with almonds and serve immediately. Bon appétit!

Bulgur Muffins with Raisins

(Ready in about 20 minutes | Servings 6)

Per serving : Calories: 306; Fat: 12.1g; Carbs: 44.6g; Protein: 6.1g

Ingredients

1 cup bulgur, cooked

4 tablespoons coconut oil, melted

1 teaspoon baking powder

1 teaspoon baking soda

2 tablespoons flax egg

1 ¼ cups all-purpose flour

1/2 cup coconut flour

1 cup coconut milk

4 tablespoons brown sugar

1/2 cup raisins, packed

Directions

Start by preheating your oven to 420 degrees F. Spritz a muffin tin with a nonstick cooking oil.

Thoroughly combine all the dry ingredients. Add in the cooked bulgur.

In another bowl, whisk all the wet ingredients; add the wet mixture to the bulgur mixture; fold in the raisins.

Mix until everything is well combined, but not overmixed; spoon the batter into the prepared muffin.

Now, bake your muffins for about 16 minutes or until a tester comes out dry and clean. Bon appétit!

Old-Fashioned Pilaf

(Ready in about 45 minutes | Servings 4)

Per serving : Calories: 532; Fat: 11.4g; Carbs: 93g; Protein: 16.3g

Ingredients

2 tablespoons sesame oil

1 shallot, sliced

2 bell peppers, seeded and sliced

3 cloves garlic, minced

10 ounces oyster mushrooms, cleaned and sliced

2 cups brown rice

2 tomatoes, pureed

2 cups vegetable broth

Salt and black pepper, to taste

1 cup sweet corn kernels

1 cup green peas

Directions

Heat the sesame oil in a saucepan over medium-high heat.

Once hot, cook the shallot and peppers for about 3 minutes until just tender.

Add in the garlic and oyster mushrooms; continue to sauté for 1 minute or so until aromatic.

In a lightly oiled casserole dish, place the rice, flowed by the mushroom mixture, tomatoes, broth, salt, black pepper, corn and green peas.

Bake, covered, at 375 degrees F for about 40 minutes, stirring after 20 minutes. Bon appétit!

Freekeh Salad with Za'atar

(Ready in about 35 minutes | Servings 4)

Per serving : Calories: 352; Fat: 17.1g; Carbs: 46.3g; Protein: 8g

Ingredients

1 cup freekeh

2 ½ cups water

1 cup grape tomatoes, halved

2 bell peppers, seeded and sliced

1 habanero pepper, seeded and sliced

1 onion, thinly sliced

2 tablespoons fresh cilantro, chopped

2 tablespoons fresh parsley, chopped

2 ounces green olives, pitted and sliced

1/4 cup extra-virgin olive oil

2 tablespoons lemon juice

1 teaspoon deli mustard

1 teaspoon za'atar

Sea salt and ground black pepper, to taste

Directions

Place the freekeh and water in a saucepan. Bring to a boil over medium-high heat.

Immediately turn the heat to a simmer for 30 to 35 minutes, stirring occasionally to promote even cooking. Let it cool completely.

Toss the cooked freekeh with the remaining ingredients. Toss to combine well.

Bon appétit!

Vegetable Amaranth Soup

(Ready in about 30 minutes | Servings 4)

Per serving : Calories: 196; Fat: 8.7g; Carbs: 26.1g; Protein: 4.7g

Ingredients

2 tablespoons olive oil

1 small shallot, chopped

1 carrot, trimmed and chopped

1 parsnip, trimmed and chopped

1 cup yellow squash, peeled and chopped

1 teaspoon fennel seeds

1 teaspoon celery seeds

1 teaspoon turmeric powder

1 bay laurel

1/2 cup amaranth

2 cups cream of celery soup

2 cups water

2 cups collard greens, torn into pieces

Sea salt and ground black pepper, to taste

Directions

In a heavy-bottomed pot, heat the olive oil until sizzling. Once hot, sauté the shallot, carrot, parsnip and squash for 5 minutes or until just tender.

Then, sauté the fennel seeds, celery seeds, turmeric powder and bay laurel for about 30 seconds, until aromatic.

Add in the amaranth, soup and water. Turn the heat to a simmer. Cover and let it simmer for 15 to 18 minutes.

Afterwards, add in the collard greens, season with salt and black pepper and continue to simmer for 5 minutes longer. Enjoy!

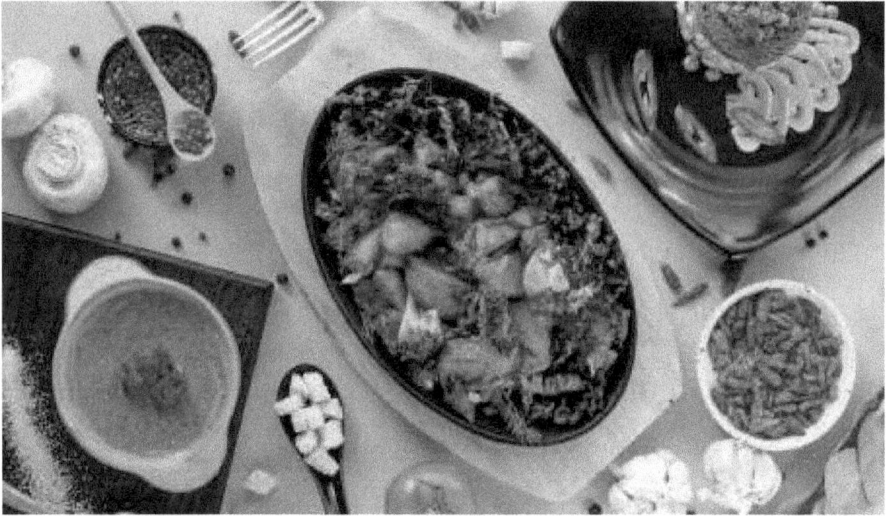

Polenta with Mushrooms and Chickpeas

(Ready in about 25 minutes | Servings 4)

Per serving : Calories: 488; Fat: 12.2g; Carbs: 71g; Protein: 21.4g

Ingredients

3 cups vegetable broth

1 cup yellow cornmeal

2 tablespoons olive oil

1 onion, chopped

1 bell pepper, seeded and sliced

1 pound Cremini mushrooms, sliced

2 garlic cloves, minced

1/2 cup dry white wine

1/2 cup vegetable broth

Kosher salt and freshly ground black pepper, to taste

1 teaspoon paprika

1 cup canned chickpeas, drained

Directions

In a medium saucepan, bring the vegetable broth to a boil over medium-high heat. Now, add in the cornmeal, whisking continuously to prevent lumps.

Reduce the heat to a simmer. Continue to simmer, whisking periodically, for about 18 minutes, until the mixture has thickened.

Meanwhile, heat the olive oil in a saucepan over a moderately high heat. Cook the onion and pepper for about 3 minutes or until just tender and fragrant.

Add in the mushrooms and garlic; continue to sauté, gradually adding the wine and broth, for 4 more minutes or until cooked through. Season with salt, black pepper and paprika. Stir in the chickpeas.

Spoon the mushroom mixture over your polenta and serve warm. Bon appétit!

Teff Salad with Avocado and Beans

(Ready in about 20 minutes + chilling time | Servings 2)

Per serving : Calories: 463; Fat: 21.2g; Carbs: 58.9g; Protein: 13.1g

Ingredients

2 cups water

1/2 cup teff grain

1 teaspoon fresh lemon juice

3 tablespoons vegan mayonnaise

1 teaspoon deli mustard

1 small avocado, pitted, peeled and sliced

1 small red onion, thinly sliced

1 small Persian cucumber, sliced

1/2 cup canned kidney beans, drained

2 cups baby spinach

Directions

In a deep saucepan, bring the water to a boil over high heat. Add in the teff grain and turn the heat to a simmer.

Continue to cook, covered, for about 20 minutes or until tender. Let it cool completely.

Add in the remaining ingredients and toss to combine. Serve at room temperature. Bon appétit!

Overnight Oatmeal with Walnuts

(Ready in about 5 minutes + chilling time | Servings 3)

Per serving : Calories: 423; Fat: 16.8g; Carbs: 53.1g; Protein: 17.3g

Ingredients

  1 cup old-fashioned oats

  3 tablespoons chia seeds

  1 ½ cups coconut milk

  3 teaspoons agave syrup

  1 teaspoon vanilla extract

  1/2 teaspoon ground cinnamon

  3 tablespoons walnuts, chopped

  A pinch of salt

  A pinch of grated nutmeg

Directions

Divide the ingredients between three mason jars.

Cover and shake to combine well. Let them sit overnight in your refrigerator.

You can add some extra milk before serving. Enjoy!

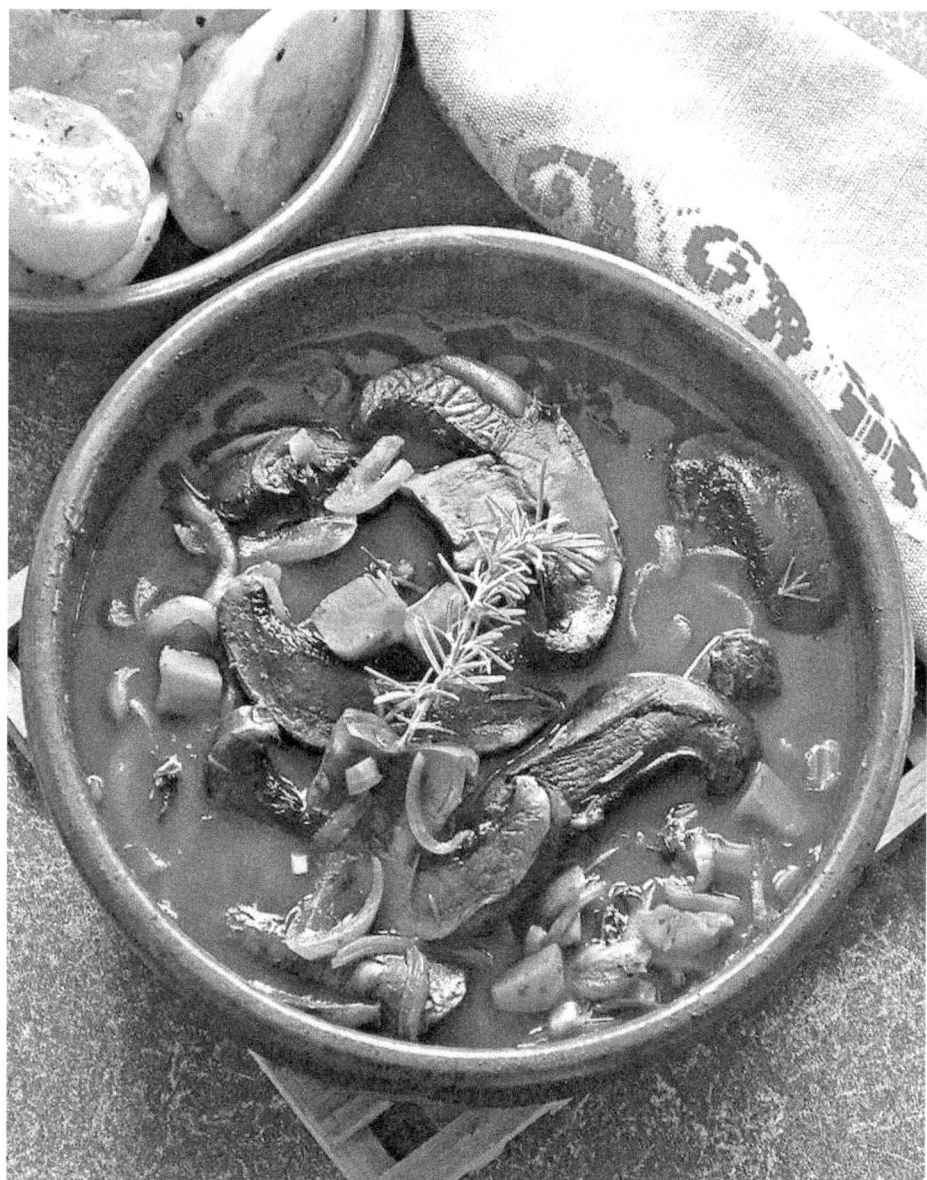

www.ingramcontent.com/pod-product-compliance
Lightning Source LLC
Chambersburg PA
CBHW060318030426
42336CB00011B/1105

* 9 7 8 1 8 0 3 5 0 4 7 0 4 *